Nuclear Medicine Imaging:
An Encyclopedic Dictionary

Joseph A. Thie

Nuclear Medicine Imaging: An Encyclopedic Dictionary

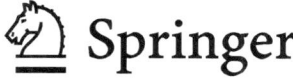

Springer

Joseph A. Thie, Ph.D., D.Sc.
University of Tennessee
12334 Bluff Shore
Knoxville, Tennessee 37922
USA
jathie@utk.edu

ISBN 978-3-642-25034-7   e-ISBN 978-3-642-25035-4
DOI 10.1007/978-3-642-25035-4
Springer Heidelberg Dordrecht London New York

Library of Congress Control Number: 2012931417

Printed on acid-free paper

Springer is part of Springer Science+Business Media (www.springer.com)

Preface

This set of expanded definitions of terms is intended to encompass those popular in planar, SPECT, and PET imaging protocols of nuclear medicine. It includes both nuclear-based scanner operations and intimately associated popular data analyses approaches. Other imaging modalities, such as x-ray, CT, MRI and a number of other modalities used in an encompassing field of molecular imaging, except for common terms, are beyond its scope – each requiring a dictionary of its own. The nuclear medicine imaging component of medical physics is intended to be exhaustively treated from a terminology standpoint. However, general biological, physiological, and pharmaceutical terminology, while also associated with scans, are not covered. These are already well summarized in various medical dictionaries, encyclopedias, and texts. A limited number of mathematical concepts likely to be somewhat frequently encountered in nuclear medicine imaging are included. Where terms have multiple meanings or can be somewhat general and generic, it is just their relevance to nuclear medicine imaging that is emphasized here.

A deliberate somewhat pedantic approach is used to explain what would otherwise be terse definitions. These include many examples. In these, the mathematical nature of nuclear imaging is deliberately kept very simple. No pretense is made to standardize any terminology. In fact colloquial usages, common in the literature, are identified as such even if ambiguous or ill-chosen when taken out of context, as noted in the Appendix.

Many definitions are based on and adapted from the authoritative National Cancer Institute (NCI) Thesaurus and Metathesaurus.[1] Effort is made when needed to orient these toward imaging uses. The author is indebted to personnel of the NCI for mutually beneficial contacts, and to Dr. Karl F. Hubner of the University of Tennessee Medical Center for helpful suggestions.

Comments and suggestions are invited.

Knoxville, TN   Joseph A. Thie, Ph.D., D.Sc.

---

[1] NCI Thesaurus, National Cancer Institute, http://ncit.nci.nih.gov. Accessed September 30, 2011.

Contents

2D mode

The property of being measured and described using two orthogonal directions. As applied to a *PET scanner*, it describes a measuring process with shielding *septa* restricting detectors' coincidences. It is generally referred to as simply 2D. Detectors' coincidences are restricted to just *lines of response* being those in the same ring of detectors. *Reconstruction* is then simplified with this directional restriction. However, there is a loss of count information due to the absorptions. See also *3D mode*.

3D mode

As applied to a *PET scanner*, description of a measuring process without any shielding *septa* restricting detectors' coincidences. It is generally referred to as simply 3D. The *lines of response* can be defined by detector pairs whether both are in the same or different ring of detectors. By making more efficient use of detectors than does the *2D mode*, scanner *sensitivity* can be increased.

4D

Denoting a process that involves all three spatial dimensions and in addition some type of time information. It can be used to designate/characterize *dynamic scan* and *gated scan* protocols.

Absorbed dose

The amount of *energy* from any type of ionizing *radiation* (e.g., alpha, *beta*, *photons*, neutrons, etc.) deposited in any medium (e.g., water, tissue, air). This designates energy deposition by the radiation without regard to the type of matter or any

J.A. Thie, *Nuclear Medicine Imaging: An Encyclopedic Dictionary*,
DOI 10.1007/978-3-642-25035-4_1, © Springer-Verlag Berlin Heidelberg 2012

biological considerations. Radiation measuring instruments, operating independently of the type of surrounding medium, indicate strictly absorbed dose. Its units can be *gray* and *rad*. See also *equivalent dose*.

Accuracy

1. The quality of nearness to the truth or the true value. A numerical value may also be ascribed to accuracy. This may be the difference between a measured value and the true value. See also *bias* and *precision*.

Example: Some *semiquantitative* analyses are performed on data from a *scanner* which has not measured its *calibration factor* for some time. In making *reproducibility* checks of expectedly unchanged *SUVs* on the same patient within a month, it was found that these are always within 10% of one another. This indicates good precision. However, for all of these an outdated calibration factor is used in obtaining *activity concentrations* for these SUV calculations. Historical records show that it is possible for this factor to vary over many months by as much as 15%. Because of this, all SUVs have an unknown bias which could even be this much. The accuracy of the reported SUVs might conservatively be stated as the simple sum of 10% and 15%, that is, 25%. This would be about the most any particular reported SUV might differ from its true value.

2. When applied to diagnoses, the fraction of these that are correct when a certain methodology is applied to a number of cases. This is a quantitative concept and calculated as (number of correctly diagnosed positive or abnormal cases + number of correctly diagnosed negative or normal cases) ÷ (total number of cases diagnosed). This measure is useful in comparing effectiveness of diagnostic methodologies in a given population composition. See also *sensitivity*.

Acquisition time

Temporal specification associated with a *frame*. Beginning and ending frame times after the start of injection completely specify a *scan's* acquisition times. When sequential frames are acquired without interruption, as in a *dynamic scan*, it is typical and convenient to specify merely a sequence of frame durations.

Activity

1. Parameter used to quantify *radioactivity* and represents *radioactive source* transformations, that is, disintegrations or emissions, per unit time for the source. Since *isotopes* are continually *decaying*, then except for rather long *half-life* isotopes, the time at which a quantifier is given must also be stated or understood.

In *scanning*, a generally unstated convention is to correct all activities (e.g., *injected doses*) to be as of a standard time taken to be the start of scan's injection. See also *disintegration rate*. Units are Bq and Ci.

2. A colloquial usage for *activity concentration*.

Activity concentration

The amount of *activity* in a unit of containing volume. In colloquial usage, this term is often contracted to simply activity when it is clear that amount per unit volume and not amount is meant. Typical units can be kBq/ml (or µCi/ml). Activity concentration is a special case of the *specific activity* concept when volume is used.

Example: 111 MBq (= 3 mCi) activity is added to a container which is to have 4 l of solution within it for purposes of future use in a *phantom* for subsequent *scanning*. It is desired to have a known activity concentration in advance in order to check a scanner's performance. This is (111 MBq)/(4 l) = 27.75 MBq/l = 27.75 kBq/ml (= 0.75 µCi/ml). Records would identify the time at which this activity was measured.

ALARA

As low as is reasonably achievable (or more concisely as low as reasonably achievable), when in reference to a *radiation dose* that could be encountered in a working environment. Brought about from encouragement from governmental guidance, this good practice entails taking whatever measures are deemed practical to keep doses to personnel working with radiation low. This approach is supplementary to various imposed quantitative limits on radiation doses that stem from health effects studies.

Algorithm

A defined procedure for achieving a goal which is often solving a problem. Its instructions can be typically implemented mathematically, which includes software executed by a computer. This includes mathematical expressions, computer programs or procedures, and flowcharts involving combinations of mathematical formulae. The goal of an algorithm is to provide a satisfactory result from input data upon executing a well-thought-out and well-defined, often mathematically oriented, process.

Example: In the example given for *Monte Carlo*, an algorithm is implemented for purposes of determining a *sensitivity* of the *slope* of a straight line fitted to its data. After performing this specific set of numerical calculations, the result shows the uncertainty of the slope that is due just to the uncertainty in one of the data points.

A

Anger camera

The original *gamma camera* invented by H. O. Anger over 50 years ago and its subsequent generations. Its principle of operation consists of a single large crystal (typically 25–50 cm in diameter) in which *gamma* rays are converted to scintillations of light. Here, a limited number of *scintillation detectors* view these through a *collimator* to provide information for an *image*.

Annihilation

Process occurring in *PET* when a *positron* from an emitting *tracer* travels a very short distance and encounters an *electron*. The result is the conversion of the masses of these particles to *energies* of two 511-keV *photons*. The latter, forming a line as they travel in opposite directions, make possible the *electronic collimation* then used in subsequently constructing an *image*.

Anterior

Denoting the front surface of the body, and thus often used to indicate the position of one structure relative to another (as opposed to *posterior*).

Area under the curve

The area between a section of the x-axis and a plotted curve representing a function. It is equal to the definite *integral* of a function between x values defining this section. In the field of *pharmacokinetics*, the area under the curve (*AUC*) is that below a curve in a plot of *concentration* of a drug in plasma against time. AUC is commonly given for the time interval zero to infinity, unless other time intervals are indicated. Symbolically, this is indicated by an *integral* as $\int Q \mathrm{d}t$ where the integrand Q in *imaging* can be a time-varying *activity concentration*. The dimensions of AUC are the product of those of the graph's two axes. It can be seen that this concept of area is a generalization of geometric area encountered if the two axes of a plot were both dimensioned as distances.

Example: A blood activity concentration curve in Fig. A.1 rises from 0 at initiation of injection to 60 kBq/ml at 1 min. Thereafter it exhibits *clearance*, that is, *decaying* away as body tissues extract its *tracer*. Sampled values are indicated by the 13 data points after injection.

The concept of an area under a curve may be illustrated by the sum of 170 small areas. Each small area is a square (not shown) associated with one of the 170 dots below the curve of Fig. A.1. Each such small square has an area of (2 kBq/ml)×(1 min). The total 0–60 min area by this approximate method is $2 \times 170 = 340$ kBq min/ml.

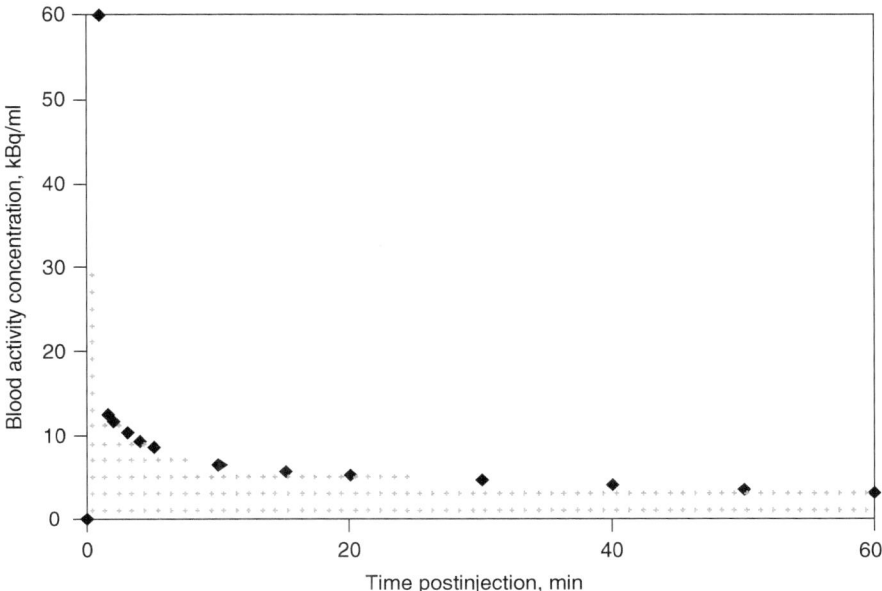

Fig. A.1 Data points along a blood *time–activity curve*. The dots are centers of small invisible squares that fill the entire area under the curve

The 0–60 min area between a curve through the 13 data points and the time axis may more readily be numerically computed from the sum of trapezoid-shaped areas for the individual 13 time intervals. Each area is (average of activity concentration values at beginning and end of the interval)×(time duration of the interval). The first such area is $[(0 + 60)/2] \times 1 = 30$ kBq min/ml; the 13th is $[(3.6 + 3.2)/2] \times 10 = 34$ kBq min/ml. The sum of all 13 is 334 kBq min/ml as the desired AUC.

Artifact

A structure or appearance that is not naturally present but has been introduced though manipulation. For an *image*, this is a feature within that does not conform to the subject and this departure being a consequence of the *scanner's* and associated software's design capabilities. Thus, a streak having the appearance of a wide scratch would be an artifact since there would be no known long sliver associated with the subject.

Asymmetry index

A *normalized* measure of a difference between two quantities expected to be somewhat similar in value when encountering circumstances of somewhat geometrical balance and correspondence as in almost mirrored structures. It is typically expressed as a fraction though sometimes as a percentage. Any of the following definitions for this fraction may be encountered:

$$(x_2 - x_1)/(\tfrac{1}{2}[x_2 + x_1])$$
$$(x_2 - x_1)/(x_2 + x_1)$$
$$(x_2 - x_1)/(\text{either } x_2 \text{ or } x_1)$$
$$x_2/x_1 \quad .$$

where relative locations of *image* quantifiers, x_1 and x_2, would also be defined. An often encountered usage is in comparing *activity concentrations* in symmetrically located left and right regions, such as in the brain. It is seen that small numbers for the first three definitions, and near unity for the last, would tend to suggest normal expected conditions.

Atom

The smallest unit of matter that retains its properties. An atom consists of a *nucleus*, made up of protons and neutrons, surrounded by a number of *electrons*.

Attenuation

A weakening in intensity. This process occurs when *radiation* passes through and interacts with matter on its way to a detector. With losses occurring during this passage, the detector receives less than would otherwise be the case. See also *attenuation coefficient*.

Attenuation coefficient

The fraction of beam intensity being lost per unit length of the transmitting material in a chosen x direction. Thus $\Delta I/I_{avg}/\Delta x$ is the linear *attenuation* coefficient μ. Here the fraction of beam intensity I lost, $\Delta I/I_{avg}$, occurs due to a small transmission distance Δx through the attenuating material. When this attenuation coefficient is constant over some distance x, the factor by which the *radiation* decreases is $\exp(-\mu x)$. The value of μ depends on the attenuating material and the type of radiation transmitted including its *energy*. See also *CT number*.

Example: It is known that 511-keV *photons* from *positron annihilation* have $\mu = 0.096 \text{ cm}^{-1}$ in water. If a detector has an unattenuated *count rate C* from a region of positron emission and then 2 cm of water is interposed, the lower count rate would be $C \times \exp(-0.096 \times 2) = 0.825C$. In the event it would be desired to determine an unknown μ from such data: $\Delta C = C - 0.825C = 0.175C$, $C_{avg} = 0.913C$, and $\Delta x = 2$ cm. The result is then $0.175C/0.913C/(2 \text{ cm}) = 0.096 \text{ cm}^{-1}$.

Attenuation correction

Adjustment for the effect of tissue thicknesses and densities through which *photons* travel from an *activity concentration* origin to a *scanner's* detectors. The *count rates* of a detector are adjusted according the amount of *attenuation* along the photon's path. This makes possible accurate *quantitation* in *image* analysis. This is because whether the origin of the photon was deep in the subject or near the surface, it will be properly represented in the final image. Information needed for making an attenuation correction may come from a special *transmission scan* of a *radioactive source* and the subject, or the use of attenuation information from a *CT* scan of the subject.

AUC

Area under the curve.

Autoradiograph

The *image* from a photographically sensitive surface or a sensor array used in an *autoradiography* process.

Autoradiography

A technique used to locate *radioactively* labeled molecules, or fragments of molecules, within a subject by recording on a photographically sensitive medium or equivalent the *radiation* emitted by *radioactive* material within a subject. This *image* produced, an *autoradiograph*, contrasts with the type of processes in x-ray radiography and industrial *gamma* radiography. These latter depend on an external radiation *source* rather than the subject's intrinsic radiation. Also, the technique is distinct from and less sophisticated than that of devices using *collimation* or involving *rectilinear scanning*. Autoradiography historically has commonly been used for sacrificed animals, as where specimens of specific tissues of interest can be readily obtained for placement on the plate.

A

Axial

Situated on or along or in the direction of an axis. In a *scanner* this axis is a line through the longest part of the subject's body. The *plane* perpendicular to this axis is called the axial plane as well as the *transverse plane* as shown in Fig. A.2.

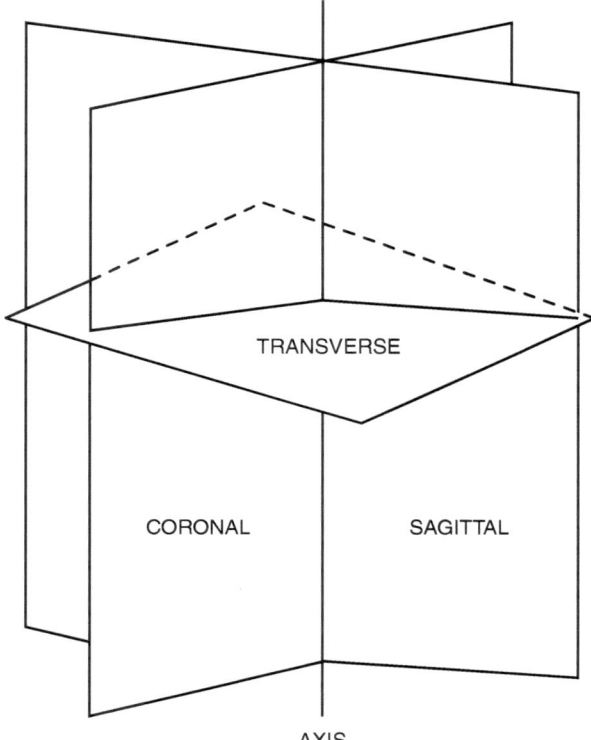

Fig. A.2 Three mutually perpendicular planes and the axis through a subject associated with these, as viewed looking somewhat down on a subject lying on a scanner *bed*. The *coronal* plane is viewable from above; the *sagittal* plane is viewable from the side. The axis is parallel to the horizontal movement of the scanner bed

Background

Existing conditions, especially those that would be confused with the phenomenon to be observed or measured. As background *radiation*, it could be an existing measure of *radioactivity* before any additional would be introduced at that location. Sources of such can include cosmic rays and prior contaminations of an environment. Sometimes the term is used to identify some quantifier of an uninteresting region surrounding a *hot spot* of interest.

Background correction

A method to adjust a *radiation* detector's output to correct for *background* effects. This usually involves simply a subtraction of a background measure of *radioactivity* from a measurement that includes both it and that from the object of interest.

Example: A counter with a somewhat constant background of 400 *cpm* gives a gross *count rate* of 10,000 cpm when a sample is being counted. The net count rate for the sample alone is obtained by making a background correction: $10,000 - 400 = 9,600$ cpm.

Backprojection

Filtered backprojection.

J.A. Thie, *Nuclear Medicine Imaging: An Encyclopedic Dictionary*,
DOI 10.1007/978-3-642-25035-4_2, © Springer-Verlag Berlin Heidelberg 2012

B

Baseline

A standard state or condition to which things may be compared. A common practice in *imaging* strategy is to deliberately plan a *scan* in which the subject is at a baseline condition, such as a normal condition. This is in anticipation of another imaging at a different condition expected to have changes to be studied. The first scan would be referred to as a baseline scan. When monitoring the effectiveness of a therapy or progression of a disease, the first scan in a series of two or more could be the baseline scan and need not be a normal healthy condition.

Becquerel

The SI unit of *activity* of a *radionuclide*, equal to one *nuclear* disintegration or other nuclear transition from a particular *energy* state occurring in an amount of a radionuclide during a 1-s-long time interval. SI stands for Système International d'Unités (International System of Units), with its core units of the meter, kilogram, and second. With worldwide acceptance of its units, the becquerel is now preferred over the historically used *curie* (= 3.7×10^{10} Bq). Abbreviation is Bq.

Bed

A *scanner's* narrow horizontal platform on which the subject lies to be moved *axially* within the *gantry* in order to position appropriate subject sections within the scanner's *field of view*. Figure P.4 shows the bed associated with a *PET/CT*.

Bed position

A designated location of the *bed* as it is moved through the *scanner* for purposes of positioning a desired part of the subject in the *field of view*. During *whole body scans*, several bed positions would be used. In each of these an *image* would be acquired.

Beta

Beta particle.

Beta particle

Electron or *positron* upon its emission from an *atom*. Streams of these are called beta rays.

Bias

Any systematic, that is, not random, deviation of results or inferences from the truth, or processes leading to such deviation. In a clinical trial this can be a flaw in the study design or method of collecting or interpreting information. Biases can lead to incorrect conclusions about what the study or trial showed. In making measurements, bias designates systematic error in a result beyond effects from the random errors that are equally likely in their positive and negative effects on magnitude. See also *accuracy*.

Example: *Standardized uptake values* of a certain tissue are measured in *FDG-PET* for a particular population dominated by obese patients whose body fat content is rather high. Examination of the traditional formula for calculating the *SUV* shows proportionality to the total patient body weight. The latter here includes weight also from fat which is known to have rather low FDG *uptake* relative to average body tissues. Hence, for these obese patients, the SUV is biased upward when being compared to SUV data obtained from other patient populations with fat content in a normal range. However, the biased SUVs would not result if some refinement in the weight (e.g., such as employing the lean body mass) were used in all SUV calculations.

Binding potential

A quantity used in *tracer* studies of *receptor* density in certain biological processes where this binding potential, as a characteristic of the receptor's *uptake*, is proportional to the receptor density and its affinity for the drug having the tracer. Typically such processes involving transmitters and receptors would be *modeled* for interpreting *dynamic scans*. Methods of determining binding potential include calculations from: *rate constants* measured in *compartmental model* fitting to data, *slopes* in *Logan plots*, and sometimes just *activity concentrations* of regions with and without receptors. Acronym is *BP*.

Biological clearance rate

The rate at which an exogenous substance is removed or cleared from the whole or part of a subject. In colloquial usage it can be curtailed to *clearance*. As a quantifier of *washout*, it is the amount (quite often volume) of a substance leaving a system per unit time with dimensions then as amount/min or amount/s (such as ml/min or ml/s).

This concept of clearance rate can also be applied to a *tracer* in the blood, as a specific part of the subject then entering into some other part of the subject. The product of this clearance rate and tracer *concentration* in the blood, *Cp*, is the amount leaving per unit time – but just into some designated part of the subject. Note that this partial or local clearance rate concept may be distinguished from the concept of clearance rate from the subject as a whole.

In *compartmental modeling*, as in the example of Fig. C.3, it can be convenient in describing local processes to define clearance rate in terms of a *distribution volume* (rather than just volume) leaving per unit time, the dimensions then being ml/g/s. If such a clearance rate is designated K_1 for some organ of interest, then $K_1 Cp$ would be the amount quantifier, as *activity* per unit mass, that leaves the blood per unit time and enters this organ.

Biological half-life

Time for an administered substance, with no further additions occurring, to be reduced by a factor of 2 in its *concentration* by natural physiological processes. This is entirely separate from any *radioactive* decay that may or may not be present. See also *biological clearance rate*, *effective half-life*, and *half-life*.

Blank scan

Scan without any subject or *attenuating* material, but with a *source*, present. *Quality control* checks involving blank scans may use a uniform source or a *transmission* source. Also with the latter, it is useful to obtain ratios of a blank scan and a subject-present scan for the various *lines of response*. These give *attenuation correction* data.

Blood flow

1. Indicating volume blood flow rate, the volume of blood per unit time passing through a specified location, such as a point in a blood vessel or an entire organ. Units are ml/s.

Example: A typical *stroke volume* of blood pumped into the aorta in each of the resting 72 beats that occur in a minute is about 70 ml. This results in a volume blood flow rate at this point of (72 beats/min)×(70 ml/beat)=5,040 ml/min=84 ml/s.
   If 15% of this, namely, 756 ml/min, flows to the 1,400-g brain, then brain tissue *perfusion* on average is (756 ml/min) ÷ (1,400 g)=0.54 ml/min/g.

2. Used colloquially to designate perfusion.

Blood volume

In *compartmental modeling*, it is the local fraction of tissue occupied by blood. It can also be the volume of blood per unit of tissue amount in a region. These usages in *image* analysis designate a blood volume fraction or a blood *specific volume*.

They differ from general physiological usage that designates the total volume of blood in some organ or in the entire body.

BP

Binding potential.

Brodmann's area

One of 47 numbered regions within a map of the cerebral cortex. Each is characterized by a particular cell organization and also corresponds to a particular cortical function. This map can assist in locating a *region of interest* (*volume of interest*). See also *Talairach space*.

Bull's eye

A *color scale* or *gray scale* display of *polar maps* as concentric annuli. Figure P.3 shows numerically how a bull's eye would be constructed in preparation for this display. While a bull's eye can be used for *parameters* characterizing *voxels* of any volume, its typical use adapts to volumes in which there is some approximately cylindrical or conical character.

Describing *uptake* in chamber walls of the heart would be a popular use of the bull's eye. *Activity concentrations* would be a usual parameter for plotting, but others, such as those of *phase analysis*, can also be plotted.

Calibration factor

A multiplication factor used to obtain an estimated real-world value from a measured or calculated value. The factor is therefore obtained as: known ÷ measured. When referring to a *scanner* its calibration factor = (known *activity concentration* at this *voxel*)/(detectors' *count rate* originating from a voxel) and typical units can be (Bq/ml)/(*cps*/voxel). When referring to a *well counter*, the calibration factor would be (*activity* being measured)/(*cpm* of counter), with typical units of Bq/cpm. See also *cross calibration*.

Example: A *PET* 6 l *phantom* containing 30 MBq is observed to give a total count rate per voxel from detectors of 60,000 cps/voxel. The calibration factor is $(30 \times 10^6$ Bq)/(6,000 ml) ÷ $(60 \times 10^3$ cps/voxel) = 0.083 (Bq/ml)/(cps/voxel). This factor can then be used subsequently to convert an observed cps/voxel to the activity concentration at that location in the subject.

CAT

Computerized axial tomography; computer assisted tomography.

Caudal

Constituting or relating to a tail; situated near the tail. It can be used in describing human subjects to designate *inferior* locations.

CBF

Cerebral blood flow.

J.A. Thie, *Nuclear Medicine Imaging: An Encyclopedic Dictionary*, DOI 10.1007/978-3-642-25035-4_3, © Springer-Verlag Berlin Heidelberg 2012

Center of rotation

An imaginary axis about which a *SPECT* camera(s) moves in its circular orbit. Perfect alignment exists if a nominally central *collimated* detector's *line of response* would pass through this center of rotation axis for all camera positions. To the extent this is not quite the case, measured correction factors can be applied to compensate for misalignment. Acronym is *COR*.

Cerebral blood flow

Perfusion for brain tissue. Though colloquially referred to as a flow, the concept is one of cerebral blood perfusion. Just as for perfusion of any tissue, this describes the volume of blood per unit time (such as ml/min) passing through a designated mass (such as 100 g) of the brain tissue. Typical units are ml/100 g/min. Acronym is *CBF*.

Example: See the perfusion example that gives a CBF calculation.

Cine

A display mode in which the object appears to move. This can be due to seeing views from sequentially slightly differing angles. Another type is seeing from the same viewing angle as time progresses. *Gated* acquisitions can also have their *frames* sequentially displayed to show a movie of a part of the subject that is in motion. These contrast with the usual static *image* display and can assist in *visual interpretation*. In the rotating cine display, a sequence of *maximum intensity projections* at successive angular viewing directions is displayed as a continuous looping process. The viewer is given a sense of depth perception when a somewhat transparent subject appears to be rotating as it shows only the locations and values of *hot spots* within it. The other type of cine display is quite similar to an ordinary movie. When used for a cyclic process, as in a cardiac study, *gated scan* data would constitute the successive frames displayed in a continuous looping process.

Circumferential profile

A plot whose ordinate is a quantifier, such as some measure of *activity concentration*, at points around an annulus in a *slice* and whose abscissa is in degrees. A popular plot of this nature utilizes activity concentration in a slice of myocardium in an *oblique* view, such as the *short-axis* view, where these slices contain annuli of the myocardium.

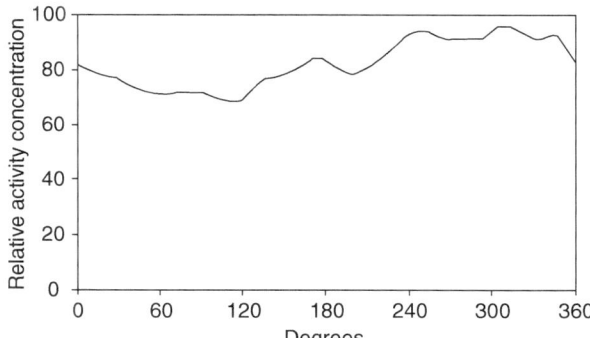

Fig. C.1 Variation of activity concentration in *voxels* of a typical myocardium short-axis slice

Example: The smooth curve through voxel activity concentrations in Fig. C.1 is a quantitative indicator of tissue *uptake* at various locations. The information in this graphical format can also be displayed as an annulus in a *polar map* or *bull's eye*.

Clearance

Used synonymously with *washout*, the process of a *tracer* leaving a tissue over time. Also used colloquially to designate *biological clearance rate*.

Clearance rate

Biological clearance rate.

Coefficient of variance

Coefficient of variation.

Coefficient of variation

The ratio of *standard deviation* to *mean*, expressed as a fraction or as a percentage. This quotient, (standard deviation) ÷ (mean), is a popular *normalized* measure of *precision*. Being dimensionless, it is often found conceptually more meaningful than the standard deviation taken by itself in describing variability. Acronym is *CV*.

Example: *SUVs* of 10 *pixels* within an *ROI* are: 6, 4, 6, 5, 5, 3, 5, 6, 5, and 5. To quantify the heterogeneity, the (corrected for *bias*) *SD* of these is calculated as 0.94. With a mean of 5, the coefficient of variation is 0.94/5 = 0.188 or 18.8%. At some later time another *scan* shows all these pixels have doubled in value, resulting in the SD being 1.88 and the mean 10. However, the coefficient of variation has not changed.

C

Cold spot

A region of low *activity concentration* within a larger region of higher activity concentration. A necrotic region can appear as a cold spot within a *tracer*-avid tumor. Cold spots do not have the popularity in *visual interpretation* of *images* enjoyed by *hot spots*. This is because of tracers being designed to give enhanced, rather than reduced, *uptake* in regions being studied. However, cold spots do play a role in *scanner* testing. Regions can be introduced into *phantoms* which have both lower (cold spots) and higher (hot spots) activity concentrations than the major part of their volume.

Collimator

A diaphragm or system of diaphragms made of an absorbing material, with open spaces defining the dimensions and directions of *radiation* passage through it. Where the subject is the radiation *source*, as in *scanners*, a collimator could be a radiation-absorbing slab of an appropriate thickness through which many uniformly spaced small transmitting holes allow a well-defined *projection* of the subject to be presented to the detectors. These are used in *planar imaging* and *SPECT*, where the detected paths of *gamma* rays from individual locations within the subject are defined for subsequent use in an *image* display. Collimators are not necessary in *PET* because coincidences of opposing detectors define the radiation path from the subject. See also *electronic collimation*.

Color scale

The assignment of a collection of hues to quantitate numerical values being represented in a *pixel* (*voxel*) of an *image*. One scale uses the order of hues in the spectrum of sunlight, with violets corresponding to the smallest values and reds to the largest. Another can be a hot metal scale where the displayed color correlates with that of metal increasing in temperature until reaching white as the largest value. See also *gray scale* and *lookup table*.

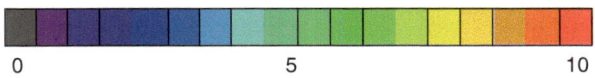

0   5   10

Fig. C.2 Color scale based on the visible light spectrum (Reprinted with permission from the Wikimedia Commons repository of the Wikimedia Foundation from file, Color_scales_for_mapping.png, http://commons.wikimedia.org/wiki/. Accessed 28 September 2011)

Example: Fig. C.2 shows the spectrum of visible light when passed through a prism. The continuum of hues is simplified here into just black and 17 others. The user of this color scale assigns numbers to the various hues, with 0–10 being chosen here. Then, an image would have its pixels using these colors to represent their values.

Compartment

As defined in a *compartmental model*, a distinct region or state for a particular chemical substance, whether at a cellular or organ level, taken to have uniformity throughout but differing from other regions or states. Thus a *radioisotope* used in a *tracer* studying a time-dependent process can be either transported (change location) or transformed (change molecular species) as it is characterized as being in one compartment or another.

Example: In the *Sokoloff model* for *FDG*, there are three compartments which allow transitions of the *tracer* among them. There is no communication between the first and third except through the middle compartment. The first compartment represents FDG in plasma before it has entered any cells. The middle compartment is for FDG in interstitial space. The molecular form of the *tracer* becomes changed to FDG-phosphate in the third compartment by a phosphorylation process.

Compartmental model

A physiological *model* of the kinetics of *uptake* involving interchanges, such as of an *isotope* in a *tracer*, between *compartments* used to determine *rate constants*, such as by fitting *dynamic scan* data to this model. These time-dependent exchanges of *concentrations* are governed quantitatively by rate constants. The latter are *parameters* which can be determined by a dynamic scan data's best fit of the model's mathematically calculated results versus a measured *time activity curve* for the region modeled.

Example: The uptake of a neurotransmitter *tracer* by the cerebellum in a *PET* study can be rather simply modeled by a plasma and a cerebellum compartment having concentrations Cp and Q, respectively. This is because there are no binding sites in this organ; the tracer simply enters the cerebellum and then returns to plasma. These entering and return rates are quantified by the rate constants, K_1 and k_2, respectively. In Fig. C.3, a *derivative* dQ/dt can describe the overall rate of change of Q as $dQ/dt = K_1 Cp - k_2 Q$. The first term is a local *biological clearance rate* from plasma that increases Q. The second describes a *decay* process in which k_2 is the *decay constant*.

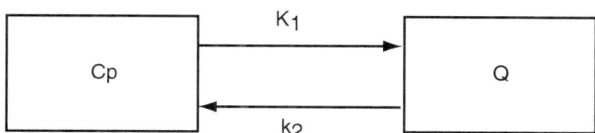

Fig. C.3 Description of a two-compartment model. Tracer leaving the plasma compartment with *activity concentration Cp* is governed by a K_1 rate constant. That returning from the cerebellum with activity concentration Q is governed by k_2

Computed tomography

A method of *scanning* a subject using detectors of transmitted x-rays, *photons*, or magnetic resonance radiofrequencies and using a computer to construct a series of cross-sectional *images* along a single axis for visualizing the subject's internals. The term, computed tomography, implies a particular *reconstruction* process that produces a series of *slice* displays in planes perpendicular to this axis. Historically, this process just used detections from x-rays but now also is applied to photon detections in scanners. Acronym is *CT*.

Computer assisted tomography

Computed tomography.

Computer modeling

A technique which attempts to provide an abstract *model* of a particular system. It utilizes a mathematical model, which attempts to predict the behavior of the system from a set of *parameters* and initial conditions. This is a common type of *simulation* in which the mathematical *algorithm* employed is implemented on a computer. Commonly, this algorithm would consist of equations whose applications require tedious numerical calculations readily performed by a computer. See also *compartmental model.*

Computerized axial tomography

Computed tomography.

Concentration

The quantity of a substance per unit volume or mass; a measure of the amount of substance present in a unit amount of mixture, particularly, the amount of solute dissolved in a solvent. The amounts for the substance and its containment can be expressed as *moles*, masses, volumes, or parts. Volume is most popularly used for quantifying the containment. A special type of concentration is *activity concentration*. See also *specific activity.*

Example: A 6 l water *phantom* has 30 MBq of *activity* added. The activity concentration is then $(30 \times 10^3 \text{ kBq})/(6 \times 10^3 \text{ ml}) = 5 \text{ kBq/ml}$.

Confidence interval

A range of values for a quantity that would contain the quantity value itself and the degree of confidence that it is in fact in this range. This is a quantity's range characterized by upper and lower limits, called confidence limits, within which there is a specified probability (such as 0.95 for the commonly used 95% confidence interval) that particular values would be found in a population of all values encountered. It is used to express statistical characteristics of a measurement result. For *normal distributions* of values, the 95% confidence interval is a range of 1.96 *standard deviations* below to 1.96 standard deviations above the *mean*.

Example: The *SUVs* for normal livers at 60 min are measured in 800 patients given *PET scans*. A mean of 2.5 is found with an *SD* of 0.5 so that the result is reported as 2.5 ± 0.5. The *distribution* of SUVs is examined to find above what SUV value there are only 2.5% of the 800 cases (i.e., 20 patients) and below what SUV value there are only 2.5% (i.e., another 20 patients). These limits are found to be 3.5 and 1.5. Hence a 95% confidence interval here is 1.5–3.5, with 95% of the 800 patients (i.e., 760) typically expected to be within this range. A simpler alternative to examining the distribution could be using a ± 1.96 standard deviations band about the mean since this distribution is known to be almost *normal*: $\pm 1.96 \times 0.5 = \pm 1$ from a mean of 2.5.

Conjugate views

Two views in *planar imaging* that are acquired $180°$ apart around the subject, such as *anterior* and *posterior* views.

Constraints

Mathematical conditions placed on some *parameters* in their determination from data. For *parameter identification* in *compartmental modeling*, this is sometimes done to avoid unreasonable results.

Example: A *mathematical model* is fit to a patient's *dynamic scan* data for purposes of identifying several *rate constant* parameters in the model. It is known from physiological considerations as well as prior model verifications that all of these parameters must be > 0. With *nonlinear parameter identification* being involved using *iterative* guessing of parameter values, the guesses are therefore all constrained to positive values.

C

Contour

The outline of a region used for purposes of delineation. It would be an enclosing boundary line in 2D (surface in 3D) that could define a *region of interest* (*volume of interest*). A popular approach having impartiality and consistency is specifying a threshold, such as 50% of some maximum, for a contour line (surface) that separates *pixel* (*voxel*) values above and below it. This maximum would be that present within a selected part of the *image*. See also *segmentation*.

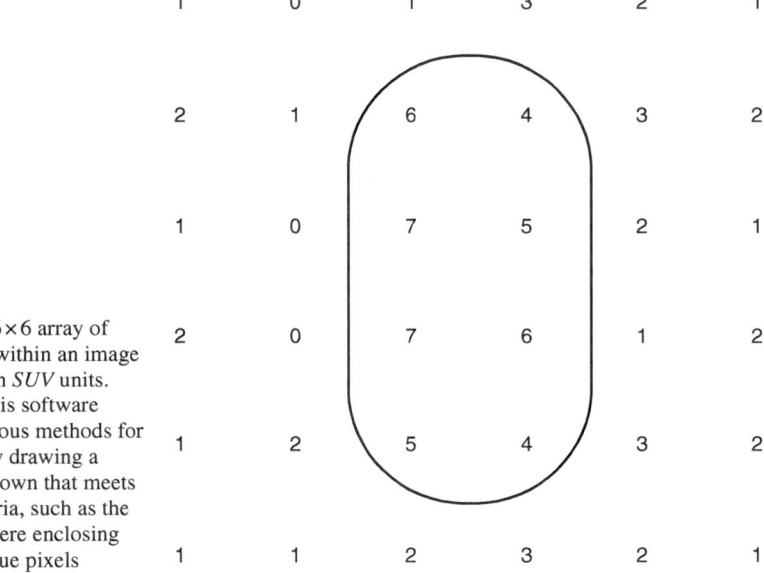

Fig. C.4 A 6×6 array of pixel values within an image shown here in *SUV* units. Image analysis software provides various methods for automatically drawing a contour as shown that meets specific criteria, such as the oval shown here enclosing the larger value pixels

Example: In Fig. C.4, the maximum pixel value is 7. It is desired to have a contour line whose region of interest has pixels above 50% of this maximum. It can be seen that the contour line shown separates values below and above 3.5.

Contrast

The degree of difference between the perception or quantification of lightest and darkest areas encompassing a region or regions of an *image* or object. It characterizes how readily a group of *pixels* (*voxels*) having an *activity concentration* Q_2 may be discerned in the presence of an adjacent *background* environment having Q_1. It can be quantified by a contrast ratio Q_2/Q_1 or fraction $(Q_2-Q_1)/Q_1$ as well as by a *normalized* difference $(Q_2-Q_1)/(Q_1+Q_2)$ that ranges from −1 to +1. This intrinsic subject contrast is unique and distinct from that of pixel brightness on the display monitor. The latter's contrast controls can choose intensity ranges of its pixels for viewer convenience by appropriate *windowing*. See also *tumor-to-normal*.

Example: A tumor with an $SUV=4$ is surrounded with normal tissue with a much lower SUV of 0.8. The contrast ratio, also called a tumor-to-normal ratio in this instance, is $4 \div 0.8 = 5$. The contrast expressed as a normalized difference is $(4-0.8)/(4+0.8)=0.67$.

Contrast agent

Contrast medium.

Contrast medium

Foreign substance administered during diagnostic procedures that allows improved delineation of internal structures by changing *contrast* within the *image*. When *CT* accompanies a *PET*, the image for the former can be improved. The contrast medium changes the x-ray *attenuation* differently in the various tissues and thus provides a means for changing the contrasts among these. An appropriate selection of the contrast medium will make it easier for the image reader – providing some improvement of intrinsic subject contrast apart from that achievable by display monitor controls.

Convolution

An *algorithm* in which one process, usually represented by a mathematical function, is combined with another performing a weighting or modifying of the function's values over its continuum in order to obtain a desired modified form of these values. This modifying function is called a convolution kernel or simply a kernel. In *imaging*, for example, acquired data as the original function might be *filtered* by using a kernel. Another example is where a *compartmental model's* output function (such as a tissue *activity concentration*) is represented by combining a kernel, having characteristics of the *model*, and the *input function* (such as a time-dependent plasma activity concentration).

When a mathematical operation is executed for a convolution, it consists of an *integration*, $\int f(x-\tau)\,k(\tau)\,d\tau$. This is often symbolically indicated as $f \otimes k$. Here, f is the function extending over a continuum and k is the kernel that modifies it at various spatial or temporal locations x as τ changes throughout the integration process. Note that integration over τ values must be performed for each x value for which a convolution result is desired.

Example: Fig. R.1 shows the activity concentrations of a *slice* through a bar as individual *pixel* values in a 2D image. In order to demonstrate here the effect of a *reconstruction* having a *FWHM* of 6 mm, it was necessary to perform a convolution. In these numerical calculations, the original function was the bar activity concentrations and the kernel was the *point spread function*. The resulting convolution was then the smeared out image shown.

COR

Center of rotation.

Coregistration

Registration.

Coronal

Pertaining to a *plane* containing a line parallel to the *long axis* of the subject's body and in addition presenting *anterior* and *posterior* views on each side of it. It is customarily viewed from its front side. This plane is perpendicular to both the *transaxial* and *sagittal* planes. An example of a coronal view is Fig. W.1. See also Fig. A.2.

Correlation coefficient

A measure of the correlation of two variables x and y, that is, a measure of the tendency of the variables' corresponding values to increase or decrease together. Extreme values of +1 or −1 for the correlation coefficient are encountered if the corresponding (such as according to time, location, etc.) pairs' departures from their *means* always have the same ratio as x and y fluctuate perfectly together or opposite, respectively. But randomness in variables results in lesser magnitudes of the correlation coefficient. The general formula for n pairs, designated as x_i and y_i, divides an unbiased average cross product by the product of unbiased *standard deviations*:

$$\text{correlation coefficient} = \frac{\Sigma (x_i - x_{avg})(y_i - y_{avg}) / (n-1)}{(SD \text{ of } x) \times (SD \text{ of } y)}$$

Example: A series of measurements on 4 subjects give results of 1, 2, 4, and 5 as x_i values. Another type of measurement on these same 4 correspondingly gives 4, 5, 7, and 7 as y_i values. This data is that used in the *cost function* example. Casual inspection shows that the second quantifier is almost always 3 units larger than the first and suggests that a good correlation exists. Calculation results show this high correlation coefficient:

$x_{avg} = 3$
$y_{avg} = 5.75$
Average cross product $= 8/(4-1) = 2.667$
SD of $x = 1.826$
SD of $y = 1.5$
Correlation coefficient $= 0.974$

Cost function

A function or expression that is either maximized or minimized in order to obtain the optimal solution or result for a mathematical problem or formulation. The cost function represents a desired effect such that its value is an optimum (such a minimum or maximum) when a *model's* best set of *parameters* have been found in fitting data. Then it could be a weighted sum of *residuals* squared which is sought to be minimized by the best choice of parameters in a model.

Example: It is desired to find a linear expression that fits acquired data points whose (x, y) values are: $(1, 4)$, $(2, 5)$, $(4, 7)$, and $(5, 7)$. This data is that used in the *correlation coefficient* example. With a two parameter expression, $y_{fit} = mx + b$, a cost function to be minimized can be chosen as $\Sigma(y - y_{fit})^2$. This is then a *least squares* fitting of data. Some results of successive guessing of pairs of m and b values are shown in Table C.1. The smallest value of the cost function, 0.35, is achieved with the optimal fitting parameters of $m = 0.8$ and $b = 3.35$. In a graph that plots the four data points, another four points, $0.8x_i + 3.35$, could be plotted and found to be along a straight line best fitting the data.

Table C.1 A search for values of slope m and intercept b that are parameters of a straight line that fits four data points by minimizing a cost function which is the sum of the squared differences between the line and points

m	b	Cost function
0.7	3.25	1.09
0.7	3.45	0.61
0.8	3.35	0.35
0.9	3.25	0.61
0.9	3.45	1.09

Count rate

The number of discrete events, that is, counts, which occur per unit time. A typical use is for a detector, where the count rate is the number of detections divided by the time interval over which these occurred. Units are *counts per minute* and *counts per second*. See also *disintegrations per minute* and *disintegrations per second*.

Counter

An instrument that can determine the amount of *ionizing radiation* in a sample. The characteristics of the instrument would be specific to the type or types of *radiation* it is intended to detect. In *imaging* where *photons* would be involved, a *scintillation detector* is commonly used. A need for a fixed geometry, good shielding, and good *counting efficiency* is achieved for photons in the *well counter*.

Counting efficiency

The observed *count rate* divided by that expected if all events were counted.

Example: A *well counter* has a 5-kBq *source* counted and finds a *background-corrected* count rate of 180,000 *cpm* = 3,000 *cps*. The latter divided by the expected 5,000 cps (from the definition of the *becquerel*) is 0.6 = 60% efficiency.

Counts per minute

A unit of recurring events expressed as a number of events per minute. See also *count rate* and *frequency*. Acronym is *cpm*.

Counts per second

A unit of recurring events expressed as a number of events per second. See also *count rate* and *frequency*. Acronym is *cps*.

Cow

Generator.

cpm

Counts per minute.

cps

Counts per second. Also *cycles per second* when encountered as quantifying a temporal periodicity.

Cross calibration

The process of measuring a quantity in two separate ways such as measuring a *radioactivity* sample in the *scanner* and a *counter*. The result is having a consistent measure of radioactivity from these two devices when both are used in a protocol. See also *calibration factor*.

CT

Computed tomography.

CT number

Hounsfield unit.

Curie

A unit of *radioactivity* in the centimeter-gram-second (CGS) system, defined as 3.7×10^{10} *atomic* disintegrations or other *nuclear* transformations per second. One curie is equal to 37 gigabecquerels. The historical origin was when the CGS system was preferred: a curie being the amount of *radioactivity* present in the radon that is in equilibrium with 1 g of radium. This is measured as 3.7×10^{10} *dps*. The preferred unit for *disintegration rate* is now the *becquerel* rather than the historical curie. Abbreviation is Ci.

Cutoff frequency

Characteristic of a *filter* that gives the upper limit for the *frequency* content that essentially passes through it. A spatial display of *pixel* (*voxel*) values may be regarded as the sum of many sinusoidal patterns having various spatial frequencies. *Fourier analysis* specifically identifies these. Such an *image* can be filtered by a type that essentially eliminates frequency components above a cutoff frequency. This is useful when the image contains a combination of: (a) objects whose contributions to pixel (voxel) values do not change drastically among adjacent pixels (voxels) but do change significantly from object to object and (b) high-frequency *noise* where small pixel-to-pixel (voxel-to-voxel) variations in values occur. The result of filtering out frequencies above the cutoff frequency is to remove much of the visual graininess associated with noise, yet without too much effect in discerning boundaries of objects.

The cutoff frequency is normally dimensioned as cycles per unit length or as cycles per pixel. It can also be dimensioned as a multiple of the *Nyquist frequency*. Sometimes it is indirectly specified by giving a type of filter in combination with a filter-width *parameter*. In such a specification, the cutoff frequency could be approximately 1/(filter width in cm or in pixels). See also *resolution*.

Example: A *PET scanner* has a filter with a cutoff frequency of 0.15 cycles/mm being applied to an image with a *pixel size* of 2 mm. The cutoff frequency may also be expressed as (0.15 cycles/mm)$\times$(2 mm/pixel)$=$0.3 cycles/pixel. The Nyquist frequency is $0.5 \times (1\ \text{cycle})/(2\ \text{mm}) = 0.25$ cycles/mm. One may also state that the cutoff is 0.6 Nyquist, that is, a multiple of 0.6 of the Nyquist frequency. A filter width described as near $1/0.15 = 6.67$ mm or $1/0.3 = 3.33$ pixels would correspond to this cutoff.

CV

Coefficient of variation.

Cycles per second

A unit of *frequency* equal to the frequency at which one complete execution of a periodically repeated phenomenon, alternation, event, or sequence of events occurs per unit of time equal to 1 s. This unit conceptually differs from *counts per second* which does not imply anything about a periodic (i.e., essentially uniform times between events) character. Acronym is *cps*.

Cyclotron

A member of the class of particle accelerator devices in which charged particles are accelerated to high speeds by electrical charges applied to two halves of their hollow container while a strong electromagnet confines these to a circular path within these container halves. Its use for *PET* is to create *positron*-emitting *isotopes*. Thus, for *FDG*-PET, fluorine-18 is produced by bombarding a *target* containing oxygen-18 with protons.

DAR

Differential absorption ratio; *distribution activity ratio*.

Decay

A gradual deterioration or decline to an inferior state, including a decrease in quantity. A type of such loss is that of a substance due to its being *radioactive* or as due to being affected by various attrition processes in a subject. It would be quantified by a *decay constant*.

Decay constant

For a quantity $Q(t)$ continually diminishing in value, the fraction being lost per unit time, namely, $\Delta Q/Q_{avg}/\Delta t$. Here $\Delta Q/Q_{avg}$ is the fractional loss which occurred over a small time Δt. When a decay constant λ is unchanged over time as is often the case, then $Q(t)$ is proportional to $\exp(-\lambda t)$. The magnitude of the decay constant λ is $0.6931 \div (half\text{-}life)$. See also *mean life*.

Example: The half-life of the fluorine-18 in *FDG* is 109.8 min. Its decay constant is $0.6931/109.8 = 0.00631$ min^{-1}. The mean life is $1/0.00631 = 158$ min here and is the time to achieve a factor of $1/e = 1/2.718 = 0.368$ loss of quantity. This is all consistent with a time behavior of fluorine-18 having a proportionality to $\exp(-0.00631t)$ with the time t being expressed in minutes.

J.A. Thie, *Nuclear Medicine Imaging: An Encyclopedic Dictionary*,
DOI 10.1007/978-3-642-25035-4_4, © Springer-Verlag Berlin Heidelberg 2012

Derivative

The rate of change of a function y with respect to an independent variable x. Graphically, if y is plotted against x, this is the *slope* measured by the quotient $\Delta y / \Delta x$ of two small increments in values along a plot line or curve at a selected location. The derivative is designated as dy/dx. Either an analytical expression or a numerical result can be called a derivative. A common occurrence of derivatives in *imaging* data analyses is in the analytical equations used to describe physiological *models* of *tracer uptake*. This is because rates of change of quantities are being described.

DICOM

A comprehensive set of standards for communications between medical *imaging* devices, including handling, storing, and transmitting information in medical imaging. It includes a file format definition and a network communication protocol. The acronym represents digital imaging and communications in medicine. The DICOM standard is kept under the auspices of the American College of Radiology and the *National Electrical Manufacturers Association.* Various types and especially brands of equipment with associated software that may interchange (via networks or removable media) image data when DICOM standards are used include: *scanners*, servers/storage, computer workstation equipment, and network hardware. In particular, *PET*, *SPECT*, and *gamma cameras* are among devices where the manufacturers advantageously use the DICOM standard.

Defining the format of the image, being a principal type of object, in some detail is only one of the DICOM features. Patient information and data acquisition details may also be permanently associated with the image as part of its file header. A special command language is available to the user for versatile manipulation of objects among devices they use. Due to diversity in the latter, it is quite convenient to have a DICOM standard.

Differential absorption ratio

A term sometimes historically used for the *standardized uptake value*. Acronym is *DAR*.

Differential uptake ratio

A term sometimes historically used for the *standardized uptake value*. Acronym is *DUR*.

Diffuse

Widely spread; not localized or confined. As used in *visual interpretation*, a diffuse structure in an *image* is one characterized by a somewhat cloudy appearance and possibly without well-defined boundaries. This would contrast with a structure having quite uniform *pixel* (or *voxel*) values up to its easily visualized boundary.

Disintegration constant

Decay constant.

Disintegration rate

The number of *radioactive* transformations per unit time and expressed as *disintegrations per minute* or *disintegrations per second*. It is the unit of measure for quantities of a *radionuclide*. Thus a quantity of one *becquerel* would have one disintegration per second. In measurements, the term disintegration is colloquially used to designate any type of radioactive transformation that leads to a detectable event. This includes a breaking apart involving a particle emission as well as merely a transition between two *nuclear energy* states leading to a *gamma* emission. See also *activity* and *decay constant*.

Disintegrations per minute

A unit of *radioactive decay* expressed in *atoms* of radioactive material that decay over a period of time equal to 60 s. Acronym is *dpm*. See also *disintegration rate*.

Disintegrations per second

A unit of *radioactive decay* expressed in *atoms* of radioactive material that decay over a period of time equal to 1 s. Acronym is *dps*. See also *disintegration rate.*

Distal

Situated farthest from a point of attachment or origin, as of a limb or bone; or directed away from the midline or midplane of the body (as opposed to *proximal*).

Distribution

Statistical distribution.

Distribution activity ratio

Term sometimes historically used for the *standardized uptake value*. Acronym is *DAR*.

Distribution function

Probability distribution.

Distribution volume

The apparent volume occupied by an exogenous compound after it is administered to an organism. This value assumes that the compound is uniformly distributed in all or part of the body of the organism at the *concentration* found in its plasma. This quantitatively corresponds to a quotient, (a tissue *concentration*) ÷ (plasma concentration). This definition can be useful when there is equilibrium between tissue and plasma concentrations. It can be a reasonable *normalization* of a tissue *uptake* that depends directly on the available *tracer* in plasma.

The distribution volume is dimensionless when a tissue *activity concentration* (such as kBq/ml) is divided by a plasma activity concentration having the same units. But if tissue *specific activity* (such as kBq/g) were used with plasma volumetric concentration (such as kBq/ml), then the distribution volume would be dimensioned as ml/g. When the tissue density is 1 g/ml, the numerical value will be the same in both instances.

Dimensionless distribution volumes having small (or large) values well below (or above) 1 indicate a tissue's relative inability (or ability) to accept tracer out of plasma. A lower limit on the distribution volume is the volume fraction of the blood vessel system within the tissue. This lower limit exists when there are no other processes by which the *radioisotope* can reside in the tissue in any form. See also *specific volume*.

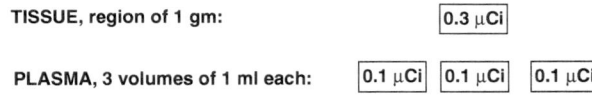

TISSUE, region of 1 gm: `0.3 μCi`

PLASMA, 3 volumes of 1 ml each: `0.1 μCi` `0.1 μCi` `0.1 μCi`

Fig. D.1 The presence of 0.3 μCi in 1 g of tissue being shown equivalent to the presence of three separate volumes of 0.1 μCi each in plasma where there is a 0.1 μCi/ml activity concentration

Example: A 0.3-µCi/g specific activity is measured within a *region of interest*. At this time, the plasma activity concentration is 0.1 µCi/ml. The distribution volume of the tracer in this tissue is therefore (0.3 µCi/g)/(0.1 µCi/ml) = 3 ml/g. This apparent volume may be envisioned as shown on Fig. D.1. A physical presence of 0.3 µCi is the same whether considering a single tissue volume or three blood volumes. The tissue is able to pack three times as much *activity* as blood in the same volume due to its *uptake* process.

Dorsal

Pertaining to the back or upper surface of the body (as opposed to *ventral*).

Dose

1. A quantity of an agent (such as substance) administered, taken, or absorbed at one time. This administration of a substance, such as a *tracer*, is characterized by the amount, such as *activity*, injected into the *scanned* subject, that is, an *injected dose*.
2. A curtailment of *absorbed dose* and thus a measure of the time *integrated* effect of *energy* deposition per unit mass by *ionizing radiation* in tissue. Units are *gray* (Gy) and *rad*.
3. A curtailment of a biologically *equivalent dose* and thus the absorbed dose times a *quality factor* which adjusts it for the relative biological damage by the type of ionizing radiation. Additionally, an adjustment can be made for *radiation* distribution among variously affected tissues. Units are the *sievert* (Sv) and *rem*.

Dose calibrator

Device which quantifies an amount of *radioactive* substance that can be placed within. It would give the number of *becquerels* or *curies* present at a particular noted time. It typically consists of a well-type chamber configured with an interior cavity that detects the *activity* such as in a vial or syringe placed within. The dose calibrator is able to give reliable absolute activities because it previously has been calibrated itself and accounts for differing *radiation* characteristics among *radionuclides*. See also *well counter*.

Dose equivalent

Equivalent dose.

Dose rate

The amount of a *dose* that is administered or received per unit time. Thus, in the case of *radiation* doses, this would be the number of *roentgen*, *grays*, or *sieverts* per unit time. See also *survey meter*.

dpm

Disintegrations per minute.

dps

Disintegrations per second.

Dual-time scan

A *scan* which acquires two acquisitions of the same regions some time apart. The first might be perhaps not too long after early occurring physiological processes have somewhat equilibrated, and a later acquisition could be after slowly occurring processes affecting *uptake* have taken place.

Example: In *FDG-PET* oncology studies, dual-time scans are sometimes performed where it is felt that a second acquisition, in addition, could be useful beyond the usual *imaging* at about 1 h *postinjection*. The second scan at perhaps 2 h uses the same *bed position* and patient location as the first and the same *region of interest*. If Q_1 and Q_2 are the first and second tumor *activity concentrations*, the ratio Q_2/Q_1 or a percent as $100 \times (Q_2 - Q_1)/Q_1$ may be markers. The larger percentages tend to be associated with the more aggressive tumors, whereas small and negative values can be associated with benign/normal tissue.

DUR

Differential uptake ratio.

Dynamic range

The largest difference between, or ratio of, an instrument's or method's highest and lowest value in a set of these. It can be either a capability or can be actual data encountered. This latter could be for example *pixel* (*voxel*) values in an *image*. See also *window*.

Example: A *PET* study is being done to compare two different protocols for measurement capabilities for assessing the heterogeneity of voxels within a large tumor. The same *VOIs* are used throughout the tumor volume in each of two scans. Results from one protocol are *SUVs* ranging from 0.5 to 8. Results from the other range from 1.5 to 9. Using ratios to measure dynamic range, the first has $8 \div 0.5 = 16$, and the second has $9 \div 1.5 = 6$. It would be concluded that the first could be favored for studying heterogeneity.

Dynamic scan

Scan having a number of sequential *frames*. Average *activity concentrations* in *regions (volumes) of interest* for the midtimes of these frames can be used for plotting a *time activity curve* and for *parameter identification* in a physiological *model*.

Example: In planning a typical *FDG-PET* dynamic scan, the beginning and end times of frames are chosen so that percentage changes of activity concentrations during the frames are not excessively large within these. This tends to a selection of shorter frame durations for the earlier portions of the scan. Additionally frame durations are chosen to be long enough so that statistical uncertainties due to the number of detections in planned *ROIs* or *VOIs* are not excessive. The goal is to obtain a reasonable representation of time activity curves from data points that are average activity concentrations during frames. A more or less representative dynamic scan lasting 1 h would be the following series that is designated by (no. of frames) × (frame duration in min): 6×0.5, 7×1, 10×2, and 6×5.

EDV

End diastolic volume.

Effective half-life

Time for the amount of *radioactivity* in a living organism to be reduced to half of its value existing at an earlier initial time. The amount diminishes due to two concurrent processes: *radioactive decay* and *clearance* from the system. If just the former occurs, this effective *half-life* is independent of initial time and is equal to the *isotope's* half-life. When there is *biological clearance* of a substance, there is also its associated half-life. But this process can be complex, and the half-life can even depend on when it is measured. Both radioactive decay and biological clearance can also occur together. Then the expected half-life for the observed *radiation* can be computed from knowing *decay constants* of the radioactive decay and of the biological clearance:

$$\text{Effective half-life} = 0.6931 \div (\text{sum of the 2 decay constants})$$

where each decay constant in the sum is $0.6931 \div (\text{half-life})$. A decaying process having a *biological half-life* can be observed directly when following the usual practice of correcting detections for associated radioactive decay.

Example: A carbon-containing drug has a biological half-life which is 10 h for measurements initiated a few hours after administration. It is used in a *PET* study by *labeling* it with carbon-11 having a 20.4-min half-life. The decay constants for the two processes are $0.6931 \div (600 \text{ min}) = 0.001155 \text{ min}^{-1}$ and $0.6931 \div (20.4 \text{ min}) = 0.0340 \text{ min}^{-1}$. The effective half-life for the observed *radiation* is $0.6931 \div (0.001155 + 0.0340) = 19.7 \text{ min}$.

J.A. Thie, *Nuclear Medicine Imaging: An Encyclopedic Dictionary*,
DOI 10.1007/978-3-642-25035-4_5, © Springer-Verlag Berlin Heidelberg 2012

Ejection fraction

A measure of how much blood a ventricle of the heart pumps out with each contraction. With each beat, a normal heart ejects about one-half to two-thirds of the blood in its left ventricle. Quantitatively, this is the fraction of the *end diastolic volume* that is pumped from a ventricle (usually the left) in one cardiac cycle. It can be measured from *imaged* blood pool volumes within the endocardial surface, as obtained from a *gated scan*. Expressed as a percent it is:

$$100 \times \frac{(\text{end diastolic volume} - end\ systolic\ volume = stroke\ volume)}{\text{end diastolic volume}}$$

Example: A *SPECT* study has built-in software to determine automatically the interior boundary of the left ventricle from the differing local *activity concentrations* of the blood interior and the surrounding myocardium and ventricular septum. This boundary is used to determine the number of *voxels* within, this then being multiplied by a voxel volume. The largest and smallest volumes when doing this for the *gates* in the cardiac cycle are $EDV = 120$ ml and $ESV = 50$ ml. These values also appear in the *volume curve* of Fig. V.1. The stroke volume is therefore $120 - 50 = 70$ ml. Hence ejection fraction $= 100 \times 70/120 = 58\%$.

Electron

Stable elementary particle having the smallest known negative charge present in all elements as a constituent in a shell around the *nucleus*. The numbers, *energies*, and arrangement of electrons around *nuclei* determine the chemical identities of elements. Beams of electrons are called cathode rays or *beta* rays when from an x-ray tube or being a by-product of nuclear *decay* respectively. A beam of electrons striking a target creates the x-rays used in a *CT scan*. The *positron* encountered in *PET* is the complementary particle to the electron, having the same mass but being positively charged instead.

Electron volt

The *energy* associated when an *electron* moves through an electrical potential of 1 V in a vacuum. It is equivalent to 1.602×10^{-19} J. Though defined in terms of an electron, this energy unit is applicable elsewhere as well. Traditionally in *nuclear* physics, this unit is used to quantify the energy of single individual particles of various types of *radiation*. Acronym is *eV*.

Example: When a *positron* and electron *annihilate* each other, two *photons* are emitted. Each has 511 keV and deposits this *energy* upon arrival at a detector.

Electronic collimation

The use of paths of a pair of *photons* traveling in opposite directions and giving a coincidence event in detectors 180° apart in a *PET scanner* to define a *line of response* along which lies the location of the *radiation*-emitting *tracer*. This differs from the use of slab *collimators* whose many holes define lines of response for *planar imaging* and *SPECT*. In PET, a *positron* (within ~1 mm of the location of the emitting tracer) emits a pair of 511-keV *energy* photons in opposite directions when it is *annihilated* by colliding with an *electron*. The detector pair having almost simultaneous detection in a narrow coincidence time *window* defines the geometric characteristics of the line of response. This information and its number of associated detections then can be used in the *reconstruction* process.

Elution

Process of a *radionuclide* product being obtained (*milked*) from a *generator* (the *cow*). The end product here in the fluid eluded has the desired daughter *isotope* from the parent remaining in the generator.

Emission scan

The usual mode of *scanner* operation in which a *tracer's* distribution throughout a subject is detected for subsequent processing into an *image*. This can be just one acquisition period over a predetermined region of the subject. Alternatively it can encompass a number of sequentially acquired views of various regions, as in a *whole body scan*. See also *transmission scan*.

End diastolic volume

Imaged ventricular blood pool capacity within the endocardial surface in a *gated scan* during the time of diastole. See also *ejection fraction*, *end systolic volume*, *stroke volume*, and *volume curve*. Acronym is *EDV*.

Example: In Fig. V.1, the maximum ventricular volume, 120 ml, is the end diastolic volume.

End systolic volume

Imaged ventricular blood pool capacity within the endocardial surface in a *gated scan* during the time of systole. See also *ejection fraction*, *end diastolic volume*, *stroke volume*, and *volume curve*. Acronym is *ESV*.

Example: In Fig. V.1, the minimum ventricular volume, 50 ml, is the end systolic volume.

Energy

The capacity of a physical system to do work. For types of *radiation* encountered in *imaging*, energy signifies their ability to exert a force over a distance as they pass though and interact with matter. A fundamental concept of energy is its being describable by the product of a measure of force and a measure of distance.

Photons and particles of *radiation* have an associated energy. For these, it is common to employ the unit *electron volt*. More generally, however, one encounters the joule as the unit of energy.

Equivalent dose

The quantity of *radiation dose* that expresses an assumed equal biological effectiveness of a given *absorbed dose* on a common scale for different types of *ionizing radiation*. This equal biological effectiveness is achieved by multiplying the *absorbed dose* by a *quality factor*. The latter, depending on tissues and radiation characteristics, adjusts the absorbed dose for their effect. Thus, due to differing quality factors, circumstances arise where equivalent doses are the same even though absorbed doses differ. Its units are *rem* or *sieverts*.

Equivalent time

Normalized time.

ESV

End systolic volume.

eV

Electron volt.

Exponential

A function of an argument that results when e ($=2.71828$) is raised to its argument's power. Common notations used for the exponential of an argument x are e^x and $\exp(x)$. See also *logarithm*.

Example: It is desired to obtain the exponential of 0.5. This is readily executed on a calculator having the exponential function and the result for $e^{0.5}$ is 1.6487.

Exposure

The act of subjecting someone or something to an influencing experience. In *imaging*, the latter would be understood as being *ionizing radiation*. Exposure is characterized by the *dose* received. The latter can have units of *rem* or *sieverts* as well as *rad* or *gray*.

Extraction fraction

(Amount of *tracer* remaining in a tissue) ÷ (total amount of tracer that entered on a single passage of tracer-carrying blood through it). This fraction is evidently the probability of a tracer molecule being retained in a tissue once it has entered via the bloodstream. A method of measurement for an organ whose entering Cp_1 and exiting Cp_2 plasma tracer *activity concentrations* are known is to compute:

$$\text{extraction fraction} = (Cp_1 - Cp_2)/Cp_1$$

This agrees with the definition because multiplication of numerator and denominator by the same *blood flow* rate in ml/s through the organ gives the amounts of tracer extracted and entering respectively in 1 s. These are the terms in the definition of extraction fraction.

Values of the extraction fraction encountered for various tracer and tissue combinations range from very small values (with Cp_2 almost the same as Cp_1) to 1 (when $Cp_2 \ll Cp_1$). This property of a tracer for a particular tissue is one of the factors involved in its choice for the type of physiological information desired from a *scan*.

Extravasation

The leakage of body fluid or cells from the vascular system to the surrounding tissues. This process occurs either by force or as a result of a pathologic reaction (e.g., inflammation). During injection there can sometimes be an immediate presence of *activity* that remains at the injection site rather than being transported away by the blood. If this is any significant fraction of the total *tracer* leaving the injection needle, then the calculation of an *SUV* based on what left the needle will result in an erroneously low value.

Visual interpretation would not normally be affected by extravasation. This is also true of quantitative approaches that do not make use of the *injected dose*. These include *tumor-to-normal* and other ratios, as well as methods obtaining tracer information by blood sampling or from blood *images*.

FDG

Fluorodeoxyglucose.

Fiducial marker

A small foreign object placed usually on the subject's surface to facilitate *scan* interpretation and *coregistration*. This could be a small *radioactive source*. When used for coregistration, the object must distinctively appear in both *images*.

Field of view

For an *axial* field of view, the distance (along the body axis) which can be *imaged* at one *bed position* by the *scanner's* detector geometry. For a *transaxial* field of view, the distance would be the diameter perpendicular to the body axis that can be *imaged*. These two distances have been customarily used for describing the related imaging volume of the scanner at one bed position. Figure P.4 shows how the moveable bed locates the subject within the *gantry* to have a scanner's axial field of view located at the desired area of the subject. Acronym is *FOV*.

Filter

A device that removes something from whatever passes through it. This generic definition includes any hardware or a mathematical *algorithm* that operates on input data to produce a desired effect as output. The latter has one or more of the input data's characteristics modified. While a filtering operation necessarily changes the character of the input on which it acts, it still is intended to preserve the desired features of the data as much as possible.

J.A. Thie, *Nuclear Medicine Imaging: An Encyclopedic Dictionary*, 43
DOI 10.1007/978-3-642-25035-4_6, © Springer-Verlag Berlin Heidelberg 2012

F

As applied in *reconstruction*, one type of filter is used to achieve spatial smoothing (i.e., reduced differences in adjacent *pixel* (*voxel*) values) in order to reduce *image noise* (i.e., random variations in values spatially) while not losing too much *resolution* capability. It does this by having a *cutoff frequency* such that *frequency* content above it is relatively small in the filter output. The frequency content being eliminated is hopefully much more associated with noise than with imaged features of interest. In Fig. S.2 the reduction in high frequency content by the display software somewhat optimally softens the edges of the discrete data value pixels being presented.

Filtered backprojection

A method of *reconstruction* that sums individual contributions to a *pixel* (*voxel*) value from detected counts of all *lines of response* passing through this pixel (voxel). It is an alternative approach to *iterative reconstruction*. Associated with this process is also a *filtering* that removes undesirable *artifacts*.

Example: A very simplified *image* creation is shown for a crude *SPECT* where the camera is simply 5 *collimated* detections horizontally and 5 vertically. The true *activity concentration* distribution in Table F.1 is a *hot spot* at the center of uniform activity within a square region of 25 pixels. The 5 horizontal and 5 vertical lines of response have the associated sums for their 5 pixels: either 5 or 12 as shown in Table F.1. Twelve occurs only in two instances: the horizontal line and vertical line of response passing through the hot spot. In Table F.2, pixel values in the backprojected 5×5 image appear, indexed by row and column number, as summed paired values from the boundaries of Table F.1. Most pixels have $5 + 5 = 10$; several have $5 + 12 = 17$; the central pixel has $12 + 12 = 24$. The last is arrived at from the two occurrences of 12 appearing in Table F.1 summed and then this sum located row 3 and column 3 in Table F.2 according to the origin of these summed numbers.

Table F.1 A 5×5 array of a subject's activity concentrations in the table interior being detected as sums (*bold*) in row and column detectors. The parallel lines of response (invisible here), defined by opposing horizontal and vertical detector pairs, along which summing occurs are shown in Fig. L.1

5	1	1	1	1	1
5	1	1	1	1	1
12	1	1	8	1	1
5	1	1	1	1	1
5	1	1	1	1	1
	5	**5**	**12**	**5**	**5**

--------Column detector sums----------

Table F.2 Digital creation of a backprojected image from the horizontal and vertical lines of response sums given along boundaries in Table F.1. Each backprojected pixel value of this image is the sum of 2 numbers from Table F.1: a row sum and a column sum, the result being located in this image according to its row number (*bold*) and column number (*bold*)

		1	**2**	**3**	**4**	**5**
	1	10	10	17	10	10
	2	10	10	17	10	10
—Row number—	**3**	17	17	24	17	17
	4	10	10	17	10	10
	5	10	10	17	10	10

-----------Column number-------------

This backprojection however does not show just a single pixel hot spot. Pixel intensity artifacts, visually apparent in Fig. F.1, always result in backprojection without initially filtering the pixels appropriately. Such filtering would normally be an intermediate step where the detected sequences (5, 5, 12, 5, and 5) are first modified by a filtering operation and then backprojected into Table F.2. Such filtering characteristics would be chosen so as to mostly eliminate the artifact. This can be quite successful especially with many, and not just the two camera views in this example.

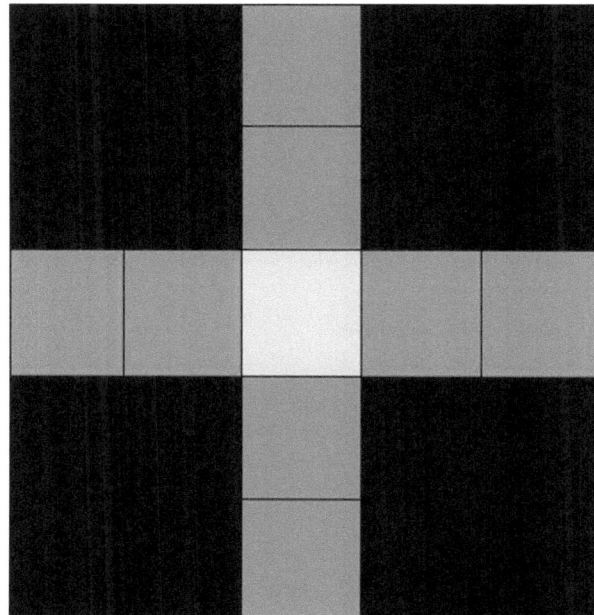

Fig. F.1 This image from an assigned *gray scale* to values in Table F.2 shows a 4-pointed star instead of a single hot spot. The central pixel suffers from a weakened displayed activity concentration due to a leakage into the rays of the 4-pointed star

Flood field

The *radiation* field created by a *flood source* for purposes of obtaining a *flood image*.

Flood image

The *image* of a *flood source*. Colloquially, these are called floods. See also *flood field* and *imaging phantom*.

Flood source

A uniform distribution of a *radioisotope* in a large container which can be placed in an *imaging* device for purposes of *quality control* checking. A uniform image would be expected if all detectors respond exactly the same. See also *flood field, flood image*, and *imaging phantom*.

Fluorodeoxyglucose

A *positron*-emitting *radiopharmaceutical* containing *radioactive* 2-deoxy-2-[18F] fluoro-D-glucose. Having similar cell *uptake* as glucose (such as high in tumor cells), fluorodeoxyglucose is not however further metabolized beyond formation of *FDG*-6-phosphate.

This *tracer* is popular in *PET* because of several reasons that include:

(a) its similarity to the physiologically important glucose;
(b) having typically *tumor-to-normal* ratios that provide good *contrast* in oncology studies;
(c) using F-18 with its 109.8 min *half-life* that is convenient for both PET logistics and studying changing cellular processes that occur before the *isotope decays* substantially.

See also *Sokoloff model*.

Focal

Any limited region within the subject which visually stands out from its surroundings. Enhanced *uptake* in a localized tissue compared to neighboring tissues would be the cause. See also *hot spot*.

Fourier analysis

A mathematical formalism that transforms sequences of values into an equivalent representation that consists of the sum of many sinusoids having different *frequencies* and amplitudes. The sequences may be temporal or spatial according to the data transformed. It is referred to as a Fourier transform of the original sequence of values. Fourier analysis is a convenient tool for use in *reconstruction* calculations where spatial data from an *image* is transformed. It is found convenient to perform numerical operations on the transformed data rather than the original spatial data.

A row of pixel values, Q_1, Q_2, Q_3, ... Q_n, at n x_i locations is represented by $A_1\cos(2\pi f x_i - \theta_1) + A_2\cos(4\pi f x_i - \theta_2) + A_3\cos(6\pi f x_i - \theta_3)$ ..., etc. Here, the A_j and θ_j are the amplitudes and *phases* of the components with frequencies f, $2f$, $3f$, ..., etc. These are optimally chosen results from employing a Fourier analysis *algorithm* so that this series accurately represents the Q_i series. The lowest frequency is $f = 1/(n \times pixel\ size)$.

Example: A *hot spot* being imaged in Table F.1 is within a row of just 5 *pixels*, each 1 cm long, and is described by the sequence of pixel values: Q_i values, being 1, 1, 8, 1, 1, are located at x_i values 0, 1, 2, 3, 4 cm, respectively. It is desired represent this row of pixel values with a sum of sinusoids. A Fourier analysis algorithm available in many types of software can be applied to these 5 numbers with their locations. The calculation output result here is a series of cosine functions having amplitudes and phase angles as *parameters* in the representation formula:

$$Q(x_i) = 2.4 + 1.4 \times [\cos(2\pi f x_i - 2.513) + \cos(4\pi f x_i + 1.257)$$
$$+ \cos(6\pi f x_i - 1.257) + \cos(8\pi f x_i + 2.513)]$$

where the lowest frequency is the reciprocal of the length analyzed, namely, $f = 1/(5 \times 1\ cm) = 0.2\ cm^{-1}$. It can readily be verified that this Fourier representation gives the 5 image pixel values. Thus, at $x_i = 0$, it evaluates to the correct value as

$$Q(0) = 2.4 + 1.4[-0.809 + 0.309 + 0.309 - 0.809] = 1$$

FOV

Field of view.

Frame

A time interval within the total duration of a *scan* at one *bed position* during which detector data is acquired for an *image*. In the usual single scan, there is only one frame at each bed position. In *dynamic scans*, however, there are a number of sequential frames at a fixed bed position. In *gated scans*, images at various time intervals within each cardiac cycle are taken. Then frame data at corresponding locations in the cycle are separately summed to increase their statistical precision over that from just one frame.

Frequency

The number of occurrences of something within a given temporal, spatial, or other type of interval. It describes repetitive rather than random events or features according to the number of their occurrences divided by data interval, such as temporal duration or spatial length. Frequency is reciprocal of the period which is the average separation of the occurrences. Thus, the concept of frequency exists for both a time series of values, such as cardiac information, and a spatial series, such as values in a row of *pixels*. The simplest repetition to identify is that of a sinusoid: the recurrence rate of its peak is an easily obtained quantifier as its frequency.

A row of pixels with regularly alternating *hot spots* and *cold spots* could easily be assigned a frequency. It would be the average reciprocal distance between adjacent hot (or adjacent cold) spots. About the same answer would result from (number of spatially occurring cycles) ÷ (distance over which this takes place). The dimensions of a spatial frequency are therefore reciprocal length, that is, cm^{-1}. It is often stated as cycles per cm as well as cycles per pixel. The latter is possible because the known dimension of a pixel can qualify it also for use when a length dimension is required.

A periodicity is obvious when a row of pixels has the values of just one sinusoidal function with one frequency. It can be less obvious visually if there is superposition, as in *Fourier analysis*, of sinusoidal functions of different amplitudes and frequencies that give the observed pixel sequence of values. Nevertheless, for the usual *images* with no visually apparent periodicity, this representation of values by a superposition conveniently allows pixel data to be mathematically treated and manipulated with certain conveniences associated with utilizing a multisinusoidal makeup.

Qualitatively high frequency content in an image is associated with fine visual detail that is displayed by variations in values of adjacent small size pixels. This high frequency content can be reduced relative to lower frequencies by a *filter* or by averaging pixels into a larger pixel size. Edges are not then as distinct. But this can be desirable when the variations in adjacent pixel values being eliminated are mostly from *noise* and would not represent the actual point-to-point tissue *activity* variations. See also *cutoff frequency*, *Nyquist frequency*, and *resolution*.

Full width at half maximum

A measure of *resolution* used when a system's response *y* (such as *image*-displayed *activity concentration*) to an ideal infinitely narrow spatially distributed input shows a *distributional* width in its values surrounding a maximum when plotted against a locating variable *x* (such as distance relative to this input location). Quantitatively, it is $x_2 - x_1$ where x_i corresponds to locations on either side of a peak where *y* is half its maximum value. For *scanners*, the system's response function would be either the *line spread function* that results from a line *source* or the *point spread function* that results from a point source. It is meaningful for image interpretation because spatial detail involving distances less than about this width becomes somewhat indistinct. Acronym is *FWHM*.

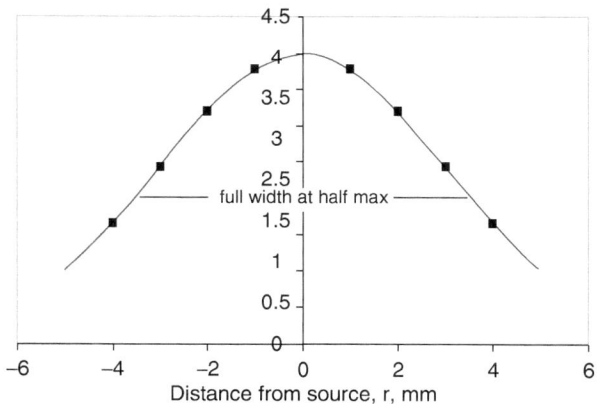

Fig. F.2 *Point spread function* obtained by an analytical function being fit to *pixel activity concentrations* (in arbitrary units) at various distances from a very small source located at $r=0$. The FWHM is seen to be 7.06 mm as the horizontal distance between curve locations when the ordinate is half of its maximum 4, namely 2

Example: Fig. F.2 shows the result of measuring a section through a scanner's point spread function. Pixel value data at various distances *r* from a very small source being imaged is fit here to an expected theoretical shape, $A \times \exp(-r^2/2\sigma^2)$, that is, that of a *normal distribution*. Data points are best fit with a value of $\sigma = 3$ mm, and $A = 4$. The distance between half-maximum-height locations of the point spread function at $A/2 = 2$ is the FWHM, namely, 7.06 mm. While this may be found graphically, an alternative analytical approach is to solve $2 = 4 \times \exp(-r^2/2\sigma^2)$ for *r* using $\sigma = 3$ mm and doubling the answer to span both sides of the peak. The solution is $\text{FWHM} = 2 \times (2 \times \log_e 2)^{1/2} \sigma = 7.06$ mm.

Functional imaging

The visualization of physiological, cellular, or molecular processes in living tissue in real time as they take place in cells. Example processes are *blood flow*, oxygen consumption and glucose metabolism. This purpose differs from *imaging* to see form and structure. *PET* and *SPECT* are among modalities that accomplish functional imaging by using *tracers* that target cellular processes which in turn are associated with some function being investigated. The term is used to distinguish the character of an *imaging* modality from that of anatomic or structural imaging, such as *CT*, where geometric relationships are a principal result. A common example of functional imaging is the utilization of brain images to study the many purposes of the brain. See also *molecular imaging*.

Fused image

Result of two *imaging* modalities after a *registration* process being used in merging these. Their superimposed images can be displayed with different colors to help show one being on top of the other. Thus a *CT* or MRI image with its *gray scale* display could appear combined with a *PET* or *SPECT color scale* image. Having anatomical detail from another imaging modality displayed along with a PET or SPECT image is very valuable to the interpreter as seen in Fig. F.3.

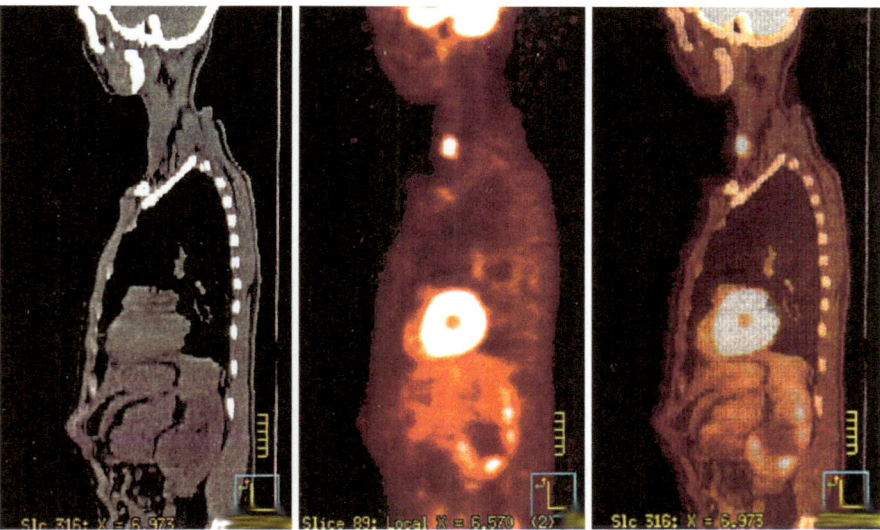

Fig. F.3 *Sagittal* fused image (*right*) of an *FDG*-PET scan (*center*) after registration with a CT image (*left*). It can be helpful to an image interpreter to be able to locate a region he is interested in relative to structural features (such as bones) obvious in the CT. To achieve a desirable display, the user can control the relative mixing of the two modalities in the fused image (Reprinted with permission from the Wikimedia Commons repository of the Wikimedia Foundation from file, PET scan image.jpg, http://commons.wikimedia.org/wiki/. Accessed 28 September 2011)

Before *PET/CT* and *SPECT/CT* devices, the modality used for the anatomical detail would take place as an entirely separate procedure on the patient. Software *algorithms* for aligning the two images consider first of all the translations and rotation angles of the subject that need to be brought into alignment. Additionally, any stretching/shrinking in various directions would be accounted for. Sometimes, this process is assisted by specially placed *fiducial markers* on the subject's boundaries that are readily identified and aligned in the two modalities. However, in PET/CT and SPECT/CT, when the patient remains unmoved on the *bed* for both the anatomical and *molecular imaging* scans, the fusion software has an easier task.

FWHM

Full width at half maximum.

Gamma

Gamma radiation.

Gamma camera

An instrument used to *image* emissions from a subject after the injection of a *radioactive* drug which releases *gamma* rays. Both *planar imaging* and *SPECT* use gamma cameras. The camera consists of a two-dimensional array of detectors. One type is the *Anger camera* using *scintillation detectors*. Here, electrical current producing photomultipliers receive light signals from gamma's from the subject that enter a special crystal. A more recent type is the solid-state camera in which the gamma's impinge on *solid-state detectors*. These have a semiconductor where the electrical current produced by the gammas is directly available. Additionally, interposed between the detector and the subject is a *collimator* that defines the *lines of response* from emission locations.

Gamma radiation

High-*energy*, short wavelength, electromagnetic *ionizing radiation* emitted from the *nucleus*. Gamma radiation frequently accompanies alpha and *beta particle* emissions. Gamma rays are very penetrating and are best stopped or shielded by dense materials, such as lead or depleted uranium. Gamma rays have the same nature as x-rays and are only differentiated by their origin. The character of gamma rays, x-rays, visible light, infrared rays, and radio waves is the same. These are all forms of electromagnetic radiation. They differ only in their characterizing *frequencies* and associated wavelengths.

J.A. Thie, *Nuclear Medicine Imaging: An Encyclopedic Dictionary*,
DOI 10.1007/978-3-642-25035-4_7, © Springer-Verlag Berlin Heidelberg 2012

Gantry

A spanning framework used to support machinery, including that for mounting any device to be moved. For *SPECT*, the gantry supports the moving *gamma camera*. For *PET*, the gantry houses its detectors and supports one end of the moveable *bed*. Gantries are shown in Figs. P.4 and S.1.

Gate

A selection of times for a *frame* based on special physiologic criteria. The latter can be from a periodic physiological signal (such as from electrocardiogram leads or respiration sensors) that triggers the initiation of these data acquisition intervals that are individually then some fraction of the cycle's duration. Frames located at the same relative times in a cycle are expected to be about the same. Hence, corresponding gate intervals in the cycles can have their data averaged into average frames for the gated *image*.

The purpose of gating is to avoid blurring that is present due to diaphragm or cardiac motion when an image data is acquired continuously over many cycles. In a certain number of protocols, this can be found to be worthwhile. See also *gated scan*.

Gated scan

The acquisition of *images* that utilize only categorized *scanner's* counts during one or more (up to all) selected parts of some cyclic process in the subject. These may be referred to as *gated* images, each of which accumulates detections from the subject as it repetitively returns to a certain position. A gated scan is used, for example, to advantage to image the heart at various times during the cardiac cycle and not encounter any significant motion blurring in each image.

Gaussian

Having the characteristic of a *Gaussian distribution.*

Gaussian distribution

Normal distribution.

Generator

A device that produces a useful *radionuclide* from a parent substance contained within. As the parent *decays*, a daughter, the useful radionuclide, is created, and amounts may be obtained from the generator as needed. The desired radionuclide would subsequently be *eluded* (*milked*) from the generator and incorporated into a *tracer*. Generators are quite convenient since no on-site complicated method of *isotope* production is required, such as using a *cyclotron*.

Example: A technetium generator has as its parent molybdenum-99 that was previously created in a *nuclear* reactor. It decays in the generator into ^{99m}Tc with a 66-h *half-life*, thus allowing use of the generator for a reasonable time before requiring a replacement. The daughter ^{99m}Tc is eluted when needed by passing saline through a column in the generator containing both insoluble parent and soluble daughter. ^{99m}Tc has a favorable 6-h half-life found suitable for protocols involving *gamma cameras*.

Geometric mean

As contrasted with the normally understood arithmetic *mean*, the nth root of the multiple products of *n* values. For a simple circumstance of just $n = 2$ values, it is simply the square root of the product.

Example: Both *anterior* and *posterior* views of a subject are taken in a *planar imaging* study, with the same *region of interest* identified in each *image*. These anterior and posterior *ROI* average values are 12 and 4, respectively. The geometric mean of these values is $(12 \times 4)^{1/2} = 48^{1/2} = 6.9$. Note that this 6.9 is not quite the same as the usual arithmetic mean of the 2 numbers, that is, $(12 + 4)/2 = 8$. It can be shown that for planar imaging, the geometric mean is the more appropriate measure to use. This is because of the manner in which *attenuation* affects each of the two opposing images.

Gjedde-Patlak plot

Patlak plot.

Glucose level

The *concentration* of glucose in whole blood, customarily given in mg/dl or mmol/l. It is also possible for this to be the concentration of glucose in plasma or serum which can typically be ~11% or ~16% higher, respectively. Since the molecular weight of glucose is 180.16 g/mol, numbers reported in mmol/l would be multiplied by $180.16/10 = 18.016$ to obtain the number of mg/dl.

Glucose level measurements are commonly performed as part of the *FDG-PET* protocol. This is because *uptakes* of various tissues can often depend significantly on the glucose level of the subject at the particular time of the *scan*. Some attempt is made to have a somewhat standard level in order to better compare scans of the same tissue. This is done by requiring fasting so at least effects of prior food intake on glucose are minimized.

Gray

A unit of absorbed *radiation dose*. One gray is equal to an *absorbed dose* of 1 J/kg of matter, or to 100 *rads*. However, for living organisms, the same number of grays can cause effects which differ according to the type of radiation and even to its relative distribution within the subject. For accommodating these considerations, the concept of *equivalent dose* is meaningful and has units, *sieverts*. See also *ionizing radiation* and *quality factor*.

Some idea of the magnitude of this *energy* deposition into 1 kg can be had by noting that 1 J of energy is equivalent to the power of 1 W enduring for 1 s. This amount of energy, such as the heat from a small 1-W light bulb, is the same as that from 1 Gy of radiation energy in this 1 kg. Although radiant heat and *gamma* radiation can be depositing the same energy here, the biological effects from the latter can be much more substantial. Abbreviation is Gy.

Gray scale

The assignment of quantitative *image* brightness levels to numerical values being represented in a *pixel* (*voxel*), ranging from white (corresponding to one extreme value) to black (corresponding to the other extreme). A typical gray scale might contain 256 shades of gray. Each of these shades corresponds to a chosen band of values in their progressive sequence encompassing the *dynamic range*. See also *color scale* and *lookup table*.

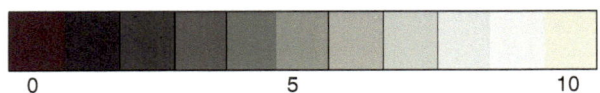

Fig. G.1 A simple gray scale in which black and 10 lighter shades are used to represent the values 0 through 10

Example: Fig. G.1 is a gray scale having a limited number of shades. The user of this gray scale first assigns numbers to the various shades, with 0–10 being those chosen here. Then an image would have its pixels using these shades to represent their values.

An even simpler application of using just three shades of gray to represent pixel values in Table F.2 is seen in Fig. F.1. The light, medium, and dark are chosen to represent ranges of values being imaged that include 4.8, 3.4, and 2, respectively, in this simplistic formulation of a gray scale. In contrast, many shades of gray are assigned to the pixels visible in Fig. S.2.

Half-life

The time it takes for a substance to lose half of its pharmacologic, physiologic, or radiologic presence. When time behavior is proportional to $\exp(-\lambda t)$, the half-life is related to the *decay constant* λ as $0.6931/\lambda$. See also *biological half-life*, *effective half-life*, and *mean life*.

Example: Some popular *positron* emitters used in *PET* are oxygen-15, nitrogen-13, carbon-11, fluorine-18, and rubidium-82. These have half-lives of 2.04, 9.97, 20.38, 109.8 min, and 76 s, respectively. For fluorine-18, if 37 MBq of *activity* is measured at a certain time, then after 109.8 min, there will be 18.5 MBq; after another 109.8 min, only 9.25 MBq; etc.

Header tag

A uniquely defined quantity appearing in the computer file such as created according to the *DICOM* standard of handling *image* data. It is important for the quantification of image features that many numerical values associated with the *scanner* configuration and protocol used be given. Each header tag is one such value.

Example: Special designated header tags in a DICOM file give information for patient name, *radionuclide* total *injected dose*, and many other scan or image characteristics. Since these header tags are positioned in the file in a well-prescribed standardized manner, varieties of software can readily access these for subsequent use.

J.A. Thie, *Nuclear Medicine Imaging: An Encyclopedic Dictionary*,
DOI 10.1007/978-3-642-25035-4_8, © Springer-Verlag Berlin Heidelberg 2012

Histogram

A 2- (or 3-) dimensional bar chart representing a *frequency distribution* where the heights of the bars represent observed frequencies of occurrence of various values. The locations of the bars according to 1 (or 2) axes associated with a horizontal line (or plane) represent the midpoints of ranges of these values. Thus the vertical ordinate shows the relative distribution (i.e., a proportionality to the number of occurrences of quantities falling within a band of values), and its abscissa, in the common 2D histogram, locates these bands. Histograms find use in *imaging* in their ability to help visualize how *pixel* values are distributed over some defined region. See also *statistical distribution*.

Example: Results of a certain organ's *FDG-PET SUVs* for a population of 200 patients having similar pathologies are categorized into six bins in Table H.1 for the histogram of Fig. H.1. A uniform bin width of 0.5 is chosen and purposely has at least several occurrences in each bin. This gives at least adequate precision in describing infrequent occurrences.

Table H.1 Data used in plotting the histogram in Fig. H.1

Range of SUVs		Number in range
Upper value	Lower value	
1.25	1.75	3
1.75	2.25	27
2.25	2.75	69
2.75	3.25	68
3.25	3.75	28
3.75	4.25	5

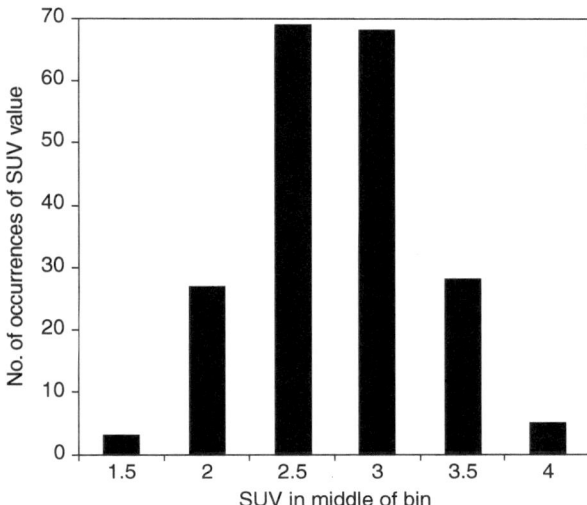

Fig. H.1 Histogram of a tissue's SUVs

Horizontal long axis

As a horizontal long axis view, an *oblique plane* through the heart containing its *long axis* and showing all four chambers. This and any plane parallel to it can be called a horizontal long axis view. These *slices* are perpendicular to *vertical long axis* views as well as *short axis* views as shown in Fig. H.2.

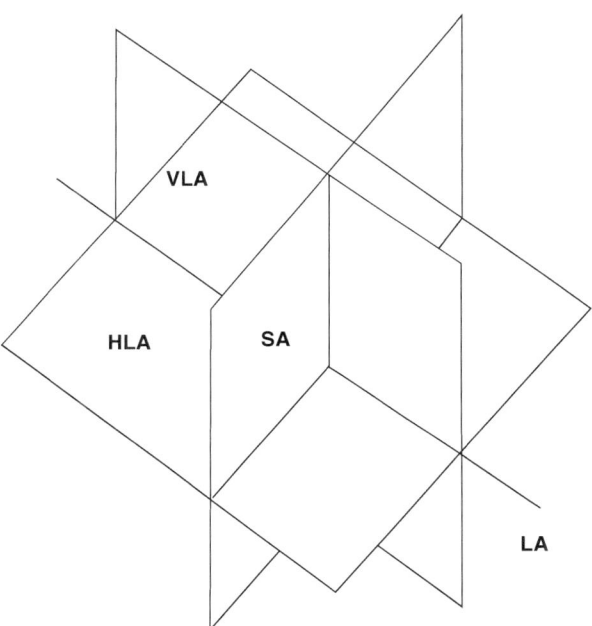

Fig. H.2 Three mutually perpendicular planes of the heart traditionally defined according to the axis they contain. The long axis (LA) passes from the apex (*lower right*) to base (*upper left*). The short axis (not shown) is any line in the short axis view (SA) that intersects the long axis anywhere and is perpendicular to it. The horizontal long axis view (HLA) and the vertical long axis view (VLA) here both contain the long axis. Planes parallel to these also are given these names

Hot spot

A center of high *activity concentration* within a larger area of lesser activity concentration. This concept is popular in *visual interpretation* of *images*. A reader is alert for anomalous hot spots yet recognizing that some normal tissue regions may also be displayed as hot spots. See also *cold spot* and *focal*.

Example: A tumor of only a few cm or less in average diameter could often have an *SUV* somewhat greater than 1 in a *FDG-PET* study. But its surroundings would typically have an SUV of near 1 or less, as characteristic of many normal body tissues. Hence, this tumor would stand out as a hot spot in the displayed image. The actual visual appearance of this, that is, *contrast*, of course depends on the mapping of SUVs in the *gray scale* or *color scale* used.

H

Hounsfield unit

A *normalized* quantifier of the *attenuation coefficient* which is *imaged* in a *CT scanner*. It is related to the attenuation coefficient μ at a point in the image by $1,000 \times (\mu - \mu_w)/(\mu_w - \mu_{air})$, where μ_w and μ_{air} are the attenuation coefficients of water and air, respectively. The resulting encountered values are Hounsfield units and range from $-1,000$ for air to $+$ several hundred for very dense tissue, with water being zero. Acronym is *HU*.

HU

Hounsfield unit.

Hybrid imaging

Use of a common *bed* for two *imaging modalities* implemented at nearly the same time. The purpose is to obtain a *fused image* from calculations more easily performed than if substantial subject repositioning/reorientation were involved.

ID

Injected dose.

Identifiability

Ability to achieve reasonable *accuracy* and *precision* in determining a particular *parameter* when fitting a mathematical *model* to data. One impediment to identifiability can be high intrinsic *correlation coefficients* among some parameters, not all of which can then be suitably identified. In such instances, *model* simplifications would be sought.

Image

Any record of a picture-taking event whether physical or electronic. It can also be the act of creating such a record. The format of an image may be quite varied and include a paper copy, a screen display, and any of a variety of computer storage approaches.

Image feature

In *image* processing, a piece of information which is relevant for information extraction related to a certain application, either specific structures in the image itself (e.g., simple structures such as points or edges to more complex structures such as objects) or the result of a general neighborhood operation (feature extractor or feature detector) applied to the image. Both qualitative and quantitative uses may be made of image features. The very act of *visual interpretation* searches for features

J.A. Thie, *Nuclear Medicine Imaging: An Encyclopedic Dictionary*,
DOI 10.1007/978-3-642-25035-4_9, © Springer-Verlag Berlin Heidelberg 2012

and details within these. A result here if subsequent *quantitation* is desired is to identify specific *regions of interest* among the image features.

Imaging phantom

An artificial structure placed within a *scanner* for the assessment of *imaging* characteristics. Within functional categories, phantoms can be further defined: (1) Body phantoms have the shape and composition of the human body or part of it. They are also referred to as anthropomorphic phantoms. (2) Phantoms that are used for standardization and intercomparison of various *radiation* conditions are often referred to as standards. (3) Reference phantoms include phantoms used to derive radiation *dose* calculations, mineral density equivalences, or other similar type measurements. Commonly, *radioisotopes* would be placed at appropriate locations within this specially constructed inanimate object to image a known configuration of *activity concentrations* located within *attenuating* materials. Alternatively, when used with an external *source*, the phantom can be employed just for its attenuating characteristics. See also *flood image* and *flood source*.

Example: A useful phantom can be a water-filled plastic cylinder encompassing a major part of the *field of view*. But it is constructed with a few locations for *hot spots* and *cold spots*. These would be small diameter cylinders respectively containing either a known *concentrations* of a radioisotope or just air. When imaged, the measured concentrations would be compared with these known values.

Inferior

In anatomy, indicating lower than a given reference point (as opposed to *superior*).

Influx constant

A measure of the rate by which *tracer* leaves plasma and is being trapped in a cell. Commonly, it is obtained from the *slope* of a *Patlak plot*, where it is the increase in tissue *activity concentration normalized* by plasma activity concentration that occurs in a unit of *normalized time*. It is commonly designated as Ki and depends on individual *rate constants* that appear as *parameters* in a *compartmental model*.

How the influx constant quantitatively relates tissue uptake Q and the *tracer concentration Cp* responsible for it may be seen in the equation for the straight line that fits Patlak plot data:

$$Q / Cp = Ki(\int Cp \, dt) / Cp + V$$

where its two *parameters* are the slope *Ki* and *intercept V*. Multiplication by *Cp* shows how tissue *uptake* is represented by a metabolic component involving *Ki* and a vascular component:

$$Q = Ki \left(\int Cp \; dt \right) + VCp$$

See also *macroparameter* and *metabolic rate*.

Infusion pump

Device used to accurately deliver a preprogrammed *dose* of a *tracer* to a subject to be *scanned* while also using a desired delivery rate. Pumps find favor because of giving consistency among *scans*, attractiveness of automated features, and reduced *dose rates* to the technologists' hands. The infusion pump is ideal on rare occasions when the tracer is to be delivered slowly rather than rapidly before significant uptake within the subject. This would be according to a specially designed function of time over a substantial duration of a scan to meet requirements of a special *pharmacokinetic* study.

Infusion rate

The volume of a substance injected into a subject in a unit time. This would typically apply to an automatic injection by an *infusion pump* where most usually this rate is kept constant. Typical units are ml/min.

Injected dose

The *activity* of a *tracer* injected at the beginning of a *scan*. Units are Bq or Ci. See also *dose*. Acronym is *ID*.

Input function

A time varying function providing causal changes to a system it acts upon. In *nuclear* medicine *imaging*, it is the time dependency of the plasma *concentration* of a *tracer*, as being the ultimate cause of tissue *uptake*. It may be measured by analysis of blood samples taken successive times after injection. Also, it may be deduced from *dynamic scans* of blood, and even some tissue, regions.

I

Integral

A summation of many products, each being a successive value of a dependent variable y multiplied by a small increment Δx in the value of its independent variable. The designation of this process is $\int y dx$. This summation is performed within limits (e.g., 0 to x_{max} or x_1 to x_n) of the independent variable. The numerical representation of this is

$$\int y\ dx = y_1\Delta x + y_2\Delta x + \ldots y_n\Delta x = y_{avg} \times (x_n - x_1)$$

Thus, an integral may also be viewed as an average value of y times the total range of x values over which the integration extends. Either an analytical expression or a numerical result can be called an integral. See also *area under curve*.

Example: An everyday encounter with the process of integration can be observed from a car's odometer and speedometer. The former's purpose can be envisioned as giving the result of integrating the car speed y as time x increases. Using only two intervals, a simple calculation showing this can be based on $y_1 = 60$ miles/h and $y_2 = 40$ miles/h, with these constant speeds existing in two sequential time intervals each being $\Delta x = 0.25$ h. The integration of these velocities over time is then $60 \times 0.25 + 40 \times 0.25 = 25$ miles. If the odometer were set to zero before the start of this trip, then it would read 25 miles and the end.

Intercept

The distance of a line or curve from the origin of a plot's coordinates to where it intersects an axis. A straight line can be described by $y = mx + b$. The coordinates of an x-axis intercept are $(-b/m, 0)$, that is, $x = -b/m$ and $y = 0$. The coordinates of a y-axis intercept are $(0, b)$, that is, $x = 0$ and $y = b$.

Example: In Fig. P.1, the x-axis intercept would be found by extrapolating the fitted line into negative x values until $y = 0$ is reached (i.e., the x-axis crossed) at $x = -20$ min. The y-axis intercept is evident at 0.5.

Ionizing radiation

High-*energy radiation* capable of producing ionization in substances through which it passes. It temporarily strips *electrons* out of *atoms* in passage through matter, thereby leaving positively charged ions behind. The types of such *radiation* encountered in *nuclear* medicine *imaging* are x-rays as part of *PET/CT*, *photons* in *PET*, and *gamma* rays in both *SPECT* and *planar imaging*. These all can have sufficient energy to create ion pairs in their passage through tissue. Ionization causes some tissue damage. This impact of radiation on tissue integrity can be quantified and addressed within the realm of radiation protection efforts. This class of radiation contrasts with nonionizing radiation where ions are not formed, as in the case of visible light, microwaves, and radio waves. See also *gray, quality factor, rad, rem,* and *sievert.*

Isocontour

Contour.

Isotope

Substances having the same number of protons in their *nuclei* and hence having the same *atomic* number, but differing in the number of neutrons and therefore in the atomic weight. An isotope can be *radioactive* or not. In the former case, it would be called a *radioisotope.*

Example: Carbon-11 and carbon-12 are two of the isotopes of carbon having mass numbers of 11 and 12, respectively. Both have 6 protons, an atomic number of 6, and the same chemical properties. The *radioactive* carbon-11 has 5 neutrons while the naturally occurring carbon-12 has 6.

Iteration

Doing a process again; a repeated performance. This can be a mathematical process involving similar repeated calculations where the results from each calculation are used to make some improvement on the next. The process generally starts with some reasonable guess for the answer. The number of repetitions, that is, iterations, needed depends on particular criteria being satisfied in the final calculation's results. It is usual in *algorithms* involving iteration to specify two criteria: one is based on the *accuracy* desired for the result; the other is a limit on the number of iterations. See also *iterative reconstruction.*

Iterative reconstruction

A method of *reconstruction* used in *PET* and *SPECT* that repeats a series of calculation steps with *image* data such that there is an improvement in the image quality in each repetition. It is an alternative approach to *filtered backprojection.* The steps, somewhat simply and conceptually outlined, in each repetition of one kind of iterative approach can be:

Start with a guessed image of values for *pixels* (*voxels*), though subsequent repetitions will use the last calculated image.

Compute all count magnitudes for detectors stemming from *lines of response* that involve *photons* from these pixels (voxels).

Compare these with actual count data for these lines of response from the detectors and obtain errors corresponding to each pixel responsible for the difference.

Based on these errors, adjust the values for pixels (voxels) in the current image.

Start the process over in the next *iteration* with this adjusted image now being an improved initial image.

These *iterations* continue for a specified number of times for which experience has shown will lead to a suitable final image. Unlike many other *algorithms* that involve iterations, it is not desirable to continue for an extremely large number of iterations. This is because each of these can add a small random contribution to the pixel (voxel) value. These random effects build up with successive iterations to become undesirable image *noise* eventually. Among popular algorithms using iterative reconstruction are the ordered subset expectation maximization (OSEM) and the maximum likelihood expectation maximization (MLEM). A theoretical advantage incorporated in the latter is making use of the *Poisson distribution* of counts in the imaging process and using a mathematical optimization technique in seeking the next iteration's starting image.

JPEG

A file compression format mostly used for digitized color and *gray scale* pictures. This standard approach was created by the Joint Photographic Experts Group to save computer storage space. This storage space can be less than required by an original *image's* format, yet preserving its fidelity. Computer filenames would have the suffix jpg when using the format. See also *TIFF*.

Kinetic analysis

An implementation of a *compartmental model* to quantify the time behavior of a *tracer's uptake* in a tissue. Prior to this numerical use of a *model*, it would have been formulated by applying the techniques of *pharmacokinetics*. Comparison of predictions from this *model* with data can allow values of physiologically meaningful *parameters* to be determined. A feature of kinetic analysis is its data requirement of multiple *frames*. This contrasts with the more usual static *scan* in which only one frame, typically acquired at some standardized time *postinjection*, is used.

In its most complete form, kinetic analysis utilizes many frames, starting immediately after injection and continuing until some judged quasi equilibrium is present in tissue uptake. Additionally, an *input function* is invariably also acquired, as this is also needed in the model, which typically could be a *compartmental model*. A determination of model parameters is based on their enabling a model prediction favorably comparing with tissue *uptake* data. These can be *rate constants* that give a satisfying physiological representation of the uptake process. See also *linear parameter identification*, *nonlinear parameter identification*, and *parameter identification*.

J.A. Thie, *Nuclear Medicine Imaging: An Encyclopedic Dictionary*,
DOI 10.1007/978-3-642-25035-4_10, © Springer-Verlag Berlin Heidelberg 2012

·

Label

An identifying or descriptive marker that is attached to an object. An application in *nuclear* medicine is where this marker is a *tracer* having a *radioisotope* and the object is a blood plasma-carrying substance.

Example: Glucose is an important substance that plasma supplies to living tissue. The carbon in its molecule is ordinarily carbon-12, a stable *isotope*. However, as a label the *radioisotope* carbon-11 can replace some of its carbon to have a tracer. This positron-emitting tracer, with a 20.38-min *half-life*, can then be present in small amounts along with the non*radioactive* glucose. However, a more popular glucose tracer is *FDG*, where the more convenient 109.8-min half-life fluorine-18 is used in an almost identical type of glucose molecule.

Lateral

Situated at or extending to the side (as opposed to *medial*).

Least squares

A popular method involving a *cost function*, namely, minimizing the sum of the squares of the differences between the data points and the analytical function (often a straight line) desired as a best fit. One use in *PET* might be fitting a straight line to data of a *Patlak plot*. See also *residual*.

Example: The three data points of Fig. P.1 are fit to $y = mx + b$, using a general notation for a straight line with a *slope m* and *intercept b*. Least squares fitting may readily be accomplished, for example, by using spreadsheet software. The pairs of (x_i, y_i) values to be fit are (100, 3.5), (200, 4.5), and (300, 8.5). The result of $m = 0.025$ min^{-1}

J.A. Thie, *Nuclear Medicine Imaging: An Encyclopedic Dictionary*,
DOI 10.1007/978-3-642-25035-4_11, © Springer-Verlag Berlin Heidelberg 2012

L

and $b=0.5$ minimizes a *residual*, namely, the sum of the squares of fitting errors of the 3 data points:

$$(y_1 - mx_1 - b)^2 + (y_2 - mx_2 - b)^2 + (y_3 - mx_3 - b)^2$$

It can readily be verified that this sum minimizes to a value of 1.5 when $m=0.025$ min^{-1} and $b=0.5$ since trials of any other values for m and/or b give a larger sum.

Ligand

An ion, molecule, or molecular group that binds to another to form a complex. When the ligand is *radioactive*, it can serve as a *tracer* and be *imaged*. Use of radioactive ligands is popular in *dynamic scans* of the brain.

Line of response

A line defined by a detector and its *collimator* in *SPECT* or by two coincident detectors in *PET*. Its direction through the subject and associated number of counts are used in *reconstruction* since it is known that the source of the *activity concentration* being detected must lie somewhere along this line. See also *sinogram*. Acronym is *LOR*.

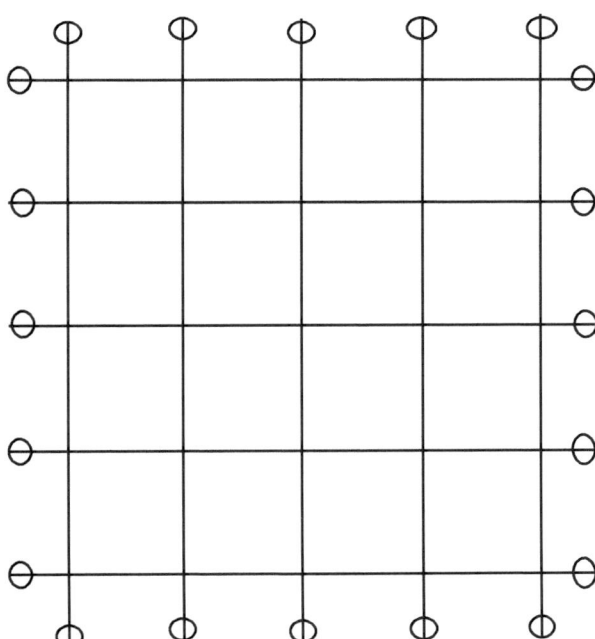

Fig. L.1 Five horizontal and five vertical lines of response terminating at detectors in a depiction of a very simplified PET, such as would be used in acquiring the row and column averages of Table F.1

Example: In PET, when coincidences occur between any pair of opposing detectors, it is known that the annihilated *positron* where tissue *uptake* occurred must be along the defined line of response. These lines are shown in Fig. L.1 for five horizontal and five vertical detector pairs. Values given in the margins of Table F.1 are proportional to numbers of coincidences tabulated by the *scanner's* computer. These values along with the directions of the lines are then used in reconstruction.

Line pair

An adjacent black and white pair of parallel lines, having equal widths, in an *image* within a sequence of such identical pairs of parallel lines. The white space of the pair has the same width as the black line. This uniformly alternating intensity of a test object producing this image can be used to visually assess the *resolution* of an *imaging* device. A set of such pairs is *imaged* as a test object and then imaged again for other line thicknesses. A minimum thickness threshold is eventually found at which the lines merge and cannot be resolved using good *contrast*. The resolution then is customarily stated as this number of line pairs per unit length that can just be resolved. In *nuclear* medicine *scanners*, a *phantom* consisting of uniform sequence of *hot spots* and *cold spots* as bars of equal width can be imaged for such a test.

Line spread function

A spatial plot showing values in an *image* that result from an ideal very narrow line *activity concentration source*. The abscissa of this plot shows relative distance from and perpendicular to the line's location. This spreading out of the line source is due to the lack of perfect *resolution*. See also *point spread function*, *partial volume effect*, and *spillover*.

Linear parameter identification

A consequence of a mathematical *model* in which all *parameters* appear as separate data coefficients to the first power in the equations used to evaluate these from fitting the model to data. When this occurs, the parameter identification process is quite simple compared to *nonlinear parameter identification*. See also *kinetic analysis* and *parameter identification*.

Example: A straight line model for fitting a set of data points (x_i, y_i) has a series of equations, $y_i = mx_i + b$, where it is desired to obtain m and b for the best fit. One approach is *least squares* fitting of this data to a straight line. The algebraic *algorithm* of this method consists of equations containing the unknown m and b along with all the known data values y_i, x_i. There are no appearances of m and b in complicated functions. These two parameters only appear separately themselves in combination with data, and they only appear raised to the first power. This is called linear parameter identification, and the equations are relatively easy to solve analytically for these two parameters.

Linear scan

Rectilinear scan.

List mode

A data acquisition approach in which detector counts everywhere are stored sequentially as values, locations, and times. This contrasts with the much more compact storage of time-accumulated counts and locations in defined *frames* having preselected times and durations. List mode storage of counts, with their locations and times, offers the versatility of being able to *reconstruct images* later with any desired timing of frames by a *rebinning* process.

Log

Logarithm.

Logan plot

Plotting *integrals* of tissue *activity concentrations* Q versus those of plasma activity concentrations Cp, but these integrals both being tissue-*normalized*. Using data from *dynamic scans*, the plot is $\int Q dt/Q$ as the ordinate versus $\int Cp dt/Q$ as the abscissa. This type of plot is found useful when at later *postinjection* times, an equilibrium is being reached between Cp and forms of the *radioisotope* in tissue that make up Q. Widely used in neurotransmitter studies, *slopes* of these plots play a role in the determination of *binding potentials* and *distribution volumes*. See also *multiple-time graphical analysis*.

Logarithm

For a specified base b, a function such that its argument results when b is raised to the power given by this function's value. Thus, for the function, $\log_b(x)$, the argument x results from the operation $b^{\log(x)}$. Ambiguity in the expression $\log(x)$ can be avoided if b is specified such as $\log_{10}(x)$ or $\log_e(x)$. The commonly used values for b are 10 and $e = 2.71828$. Usage of the latter can be indicated by the term natural logarithm, which is often abbreviated as ln and avoids ambiguity. See also *exponential*. Abbreviation is *log*.

Example: It is desired to obtain both $\log_{10}(x)$ and $\log_e(x)$ when x is 2. The results, historically found by accessing mathematical tables, are now conveniently obtained in calculators as 0.3010 and 0.6931. These answers may be checked by raising the base to these powers: $10^{0.3.010} = 2$ and $e^{0.6931} = 2$.

Long axis

Line through and in the direction of an object's characteristic feature that is longer than any other feature. One type of long axis is a centered *inferior*-to-*superior* line through the human body. In cardiology, however, the long axis would be the line, shown in Fig. H.2, from the apex center to a chosen center of the base. An *algorithm* fitting a heart model to *image* data can deduce an exactly defined long axis. See also *short axis*.

Lookup table

A table in *imaging* used for interpreting *pixels* (*voxels*) to find the correspondence between image intensity values and displayed hues or shades of gray for the particular *color scale* or *gray scale* employed. This type of lookup table is a special case of a table being used to map one quantity against another. The table is designed to give a convenient display for interpretation by the viewer.

Example: Fig. G.1 is a simple example of a lookup table. Shades of gray corresponding to 0, 5, and 10 are indicated, and correspondences for other numbers are readily found. Having this table, an image from rounded-off numerical data in this range may readily be constructed. Conversely, any image based on this table may be converted to its underlying numerical values at its pixels (voxels).

LOR

Line of response.

Macroparameter

A combination of fundamental *parameters*, such as would involve their products, sums, and quotients. The latter may be, for example, constructed from *rate constants* obtained from a *parameter identification* process.

Example: A commonly encountered macroparameter is the *influx constant Ki* which can be obtained from a *Patlak plot*. It is related to rate constants which can be obtained from a *compartmental model*, such as the *Sokoloff model* for *FDG-PET* studies:

$$Ki = K_1 k_3 / \left(k_2 + k_3 \right)$$

The rate constants K_1, k_2, and k_3 are respectively associated with three cellular processes in a *compartmental model*: influx from plasma to a free *tracer* state, efflux back to plasma from this state, and metabolism from free to bound tracer. Besides having physiologic meaning, this particular macroparameter can often have better *precision* than that of the rate constants themselves.

Matrix

An organized array or table of quantities where the elements can be indexed by their locations on multidimensional (1, 2, 3, or more) axes used in its display. The commonly encountered 2D matrix has an $n \times m$ *matrix size* which tabulates entries in n rows and m columns, with each element designated by its row and column index numbers. Special addition and multiplication rules for manipulating elements within and among matrices can provide advantages for their use when organized data is manipulated. Square $n \times n$ matrices containing *activity concentration* values with n

pixels on a side would be encountered in *imaging* a subject's *transverse plane*. The dimensional width as well as height of the 2D *field of view* encompassed by this matrix is $n \times (pixel\ size)$.

Example: A 3×2 matrix with symbols designating values of its elements M_{ij} can be:

$$
\begin{array}{ll}
M_{11}\ M_{12} & 1 \quad 3 \\
M_{21}\ M_{22} = 2 & 5 \\
M_{31}\ M_{32} & 1 \quad 4
\end{array}
$$

The first digit of the subscript designates the row number and the second the column number.

Matrix size

A quantifying property of a *matrix* that gives the total number of elements in each of its directions. For example, matrix size would be specified as 3×2 if its 6 elements were distributed into 3 rows and 2 columns. For 2D (or 3D) *images* displaying *pixels* (*voxels*), it is the description of the number of pixels (or voxels) in each of the 2 (or 3) mutually perpendicular directions. In any given direction, this number is the image dimension in that direction divided by the *pixel size* (or *voxel size*) in that direction.

Maximum intensity projection

A 2D display that results when its *pixels* are given the *activity concentration* values that are solely from the largest *voxel* value encountered along each of the lines of sight perpendicular to this *projection plane*. Various viewing angles can be chosen to generate a number of these projections. If desired, a perception of a rotating somewhat transparent subject can be created by a sequential flashing of these separate views, spaced at uniform angular increments. See also *cine*. Acronym is *MIP*.

		Top of slice			MIP line
→	10	12	13	11	13
→	11	14	14	10	14
→	13	16	18	12	18
→	12	20	14	14	20
→	11	19	13	12	19
→	11	14	13	10	14

Fig. M.1 *Voxel* values in a 6-row × 4-column *sagittal slice* being viewed from the edge of this slice to obtain maximum values for one MIP line. These values along this vertical line give one column of the *coronal* MIP

Example: Fig. M.1 shows voxel values in a sagittal plane slice through a subject. The parallel arrows indicate an *anterior* to *posterior* viewing direction seeking maximum voxel values in this slice. For each row, it can be seen that the values in this one MIP line column are the largest encountered in examining these horizontal rows. Parallel sagittal slices give other MIP lines for constructing an entire coronal MIP. This entire process may also be done for other viewing directions.

Maximum pixel

The largest *activity concentration* occurring for a *pixel* within a *region of interest*. This is a popular quantifier since it is somewhat unique for a region. If there were no *image noise* it would be quite unique. See also SUV_{max}.

Maximum voxel

The largest *activity concentration* occurring for a *voxel* within a *volume of interest*. This is a popular quantifier since it is somewhat unique for a region. If there were no *image noise* it would be quite unique. See also SUV_{max}.

MBF

Myocardial blood flow.

Mean

The sum of a set of values divided by the number of values in the set. It is commonly referred to as the average value. See also *median*.

Example: The mean of the series of numbers, 2, 19, 5, 23, and 1 is their sum 50 divided by 5 present in the series, with the result of $50 \div 5 = 10$ as the mean.

Mean life

For continually decreasing quantities, the time for a quantity to diminish by a factor of $e = 2.718$. When the quantity present has a time behavior proportional to $\exp(-\lambda t)$, then this latter is $1/e$ when $\lambda t_{mean} = 1$. Hence $t_{mean} = 1/\lambda$, that is, the reciprocal of the *decay constant* λ. In such processes, it is related to the *half-life* $t_{1/2}$ as being $t_{mean} = t_{1/2} \div 0.6931$. This is because when $\lambda t_{1/2} = t_{1/2}/t_{mean} = 0.6931$, the $\exp(-0.6931) = 1/2$.

The term originates as being the average of a distribution of many individual sequential *decay* times for a process where the totality of all these individuals is diminishing as time progresses. Here, hypothetically, many *radioactive* molecules would be individually "watched" and their times to undergo decay after a given starting time noted and then these times averaged. However, the practical approach to obtaining this same *mean* time is to make measurements of total quantities still remaining as time progresses. Times required for a quantity to decay by 1/2 or by 1/*e* can readily be measured.

Example: The *positron* emitter F-18 has a $t_{1/2} = 109.77$ min half-life. The mean life is $109.77/0.6931 = 158.4$ min. The decay constant is $1/158.4 = 0.00631$ min^{-1}.

Medial

Toward the middle or inside (as opposed to *lateral*).

Median

The value which has an equal number of values greater and less than it in a *distribution* of values. The median assists in characterizing a distribution especially when the shape of the *probability distribution* is rather asymmetric (i.e., somewhat large and somewhat small values not being almost equally likely). The median and the *mean* will be rather different or close for rather asymmetric or almost symmetric distributions, respectively.

Example: The median of the series of numbers, 2, 19, 5, 23, and 1 can be determined by arranging these in order and finding the midpoint. The reordered series is 1, 2, 5, 19, and 23. The midpoint here is 5, which is the median. If there had been an even number of values, the midpoint would fall between two numbers. These would be averaged for the median.

Medical internal radiation dose

The *absorbed dose* for a subject that results from ingestion of *sources* of *radiation* that reside throughout the subject over time. In particular, a well-defined medical internal radiation dose (*MIRD*) system of calculating this *dose* for *radiopharmaceuticals* in humans from properties of the subject and its internal *sources* has been developed and maintained by the Society of *Nuclear* Medicine. This calculation approach is quite convenient when compared to any attempt at measurement which can be complex.

Many factors must be considered in such calculations. Some of these are: the geometric *distribution* of the *activity concentrations* and *target* regions for their radiation such as organs, the *biological clearance rates*, *half-lives* of the *radionu-clides*, types and *energies* of radiation involved, and the latter's *attenuation* characteristics. The calculations involve considering for each source location many target locations. The latter's absorbed doses from all the sources can then be summed.

Metabolic process

Organic processes in a cell or organism that are necessary to sustain life. *Tracers* are developed to target such processes in specific manners. See also *metabolic rate*.

Example: A common metabolic process in *PET* is that involving the *uptake* of *FDG*. According to the *Sokoloff model,* after it is taken up by a tissue, an enzyme, hexokinase, enables the molecule to be transformed into fluorodeoxyglucose-6-phosphate. Similarly glucose for which FDG is an analog is transformed at this point into glucose-6-phosphate. The similarity between FDG and glucose at least in this initial part of the metabolic process is an underlying reason for the degree of success FDG enjoys as a diagnostic marker.

Metabolic rate

For quantifying a *metabolic process* which has been *modeled* during *image* analysis, a quantity consisting of the product of the *influx constant* and the plasma *concentration* of a non*radioactive* native substance. This latter would correspond to a *tracer* used to determine the influx constant. Physiologically this indicates the amount of the native substance that would be metabolized in a standard volume or mass of a tissue region per unit time if both it and the *tracer* would have the same behavior. Conventions for its units are both μmol/100 g/min and mg/100 g/min.

Example: An *FDG-PET dynamic scan* is performed in which the result for the influx constant is 0.020 ml/g/min = 2.0 ml/100 g/min. The plasma concentration of glucose, for which FDG is an analog, is 120 mg/dl = 1.20 mg/ml. The product of these is 2.0 × 1.20 = 2.4 mg/100 g/min as the metabolic rate of FDG. In this dimensioning, the mg is that of glucose *uptake*, and the 100 g is 100 grams of tissue.

Metabolite

Any substance involved in metabolism, either as a product of metabolism or as necessary for metabolism. When a *radioactive tracer* is used to study metabolism, a metabolite, though another substance, can also be radioactive. With its physiologic behavior differing from that of the tracer, it can be a confounding contributor to the *image* interpretation. To make use of measured blood total *activity concentrations* in

M

instances where metabolites are also present, it is generally necessary to know any significant (time-dependent) fraction of activity concentration that these represent.

Example: In *PET* studies of the cerebral dopaminergic system, the tracer FDOPA (6-[^{18}F]fluoro-L-DOPA) is used. As plasma containing it circulates through the body, another type of molecule having F-18 builds up. This is a metabolite, OMFD (O-methyl-[^{18}F]fluoro-DOPA). In interpreting the F-18 *uptake* in the brain, especially with a *compartmental model*, it is necessary to account for both molecular forms. This would include special analyses performed on the plasma to determine the ratio of the F-18 in FDPOA to F-18 in OMFD at various times.

MicroPET, micro PET, or micro-PET

A dedicated *PET scanner* with a small diameter ring of detectors that bring these close to small subjects especially some animals. Improved *resolutions* are achievable in these compared to those for the large diameter detector rings that accommodate humans.

Milking

Elution.

MIP

Maximum intensity projection.

MIRD

Medical internal radiation dose.

Model

A representation of something often idealized or modified to make it conceptually easier to understand. A special meaning would be for a system that behaves like that being studied. This system, designated as a model, may be a physical, including biological (such as an animal), characterization. It may also be a mathematical model, that is, a description (such as a set of equations or formulae) intended to exhibit the same behavior as a physiologic process. Some intents of a model are to provide understanding, permit identifications of meaningful diagnostic markers, and sometimes to predict future performance based on past data.

Example: A popular model for *tracer uptake* in oncologic studies is a mathematical one which describes tracer movement among three *compartments*. These are tracer presence in plasma, the same tracer form within tissue, and another tracer form within tissue. The *Sokoloff model*, widely used in *FDG-PET* data analysis, is of this form.

Mole

A unit of amount of substance and being one of the seven base units of the International System of Units (Systeme International d'Unites, with the acronym, SI). It is the amount of substance that contains as many elementary units as there are *atoms* in 0.012 kg of carbon-12. When the mole is used, the elementary entities must be specified and may be atoms, molecules, ions, *electrons*, other particles, or specified groups of such particles. For molecules, it is the mass of a substance corresponding to a gram molecular weight, that is, the number of grams of a substance that equals its molecular weight which is the sum of the atomic weights of the atoms that comprise the molecule. Based on this carbon-12 standard, there are 6.022×10^{23} (known as Avogadro's number) molecules in a mole regardless of the substance.

Example: In plasma chemistry in support of *FDG-PET* amounts of glucose, $C_6H_{12}O_6$, are measured. A patient has a serum glucose level of 120 mg/dl. To find the number of moles in 120 mg of glucose, this is divided by the molecular weight. The latter is $6 \times 12.01 + 12 \times 1.008 + 6 \times 16 = 180.16$ g/mol by summing contributions of atomic weights. Hence, there are 0.120 g/dl ÷ 180.16 g/mol = 0.000666 mol/dl or 6.66 μmol/ml.

Molecular imaging

The visualization, characterization, and measurement of biological processes at the molecular and cellular levels in humans and other living systems. Molecular imaging typically includes two- or three-dimensional *imaging* as well as quantification over time. The techniques used include radiotracer imaging/*nuclear* medicine, magnetic resonance imaging, magnetic resonance spectroscopy, optical imaging, ultrasound, and others. This definition was adopted by the Society of Nuclear Medicine in 2007. See also *functional imaging*.

Monte Carlo

A computing method involving many similar individual, yet randomly differing, calculations. The individual calculations differ due to the introduction of random numbers in each for some input quantity or quantities. The intent is often to *simulate* mathematically some process having a random aspect in its nature.

Example: For the *least squares* fit of the data in Fig. P.1, it is desired to know how the fitted *slope m* is affected by a random error in the measured value of the final point, $y_3 = 8.5$. One approach for purposes of demonstration here is a Monte Carlo calculation. A series of determinations of m for various (somewhat) random y_3 values near 8.5 are performed, with all other x_i and y_i remaining unchanged. The y_3 values are 8.5 + a random number. Results are in Table M.1. The desired *sensitivity*, as change in m per unit change in y_3 using standard deviations, is 0.003808/0.7616 = 0.0050. While only five trials are used for illustration, typical Monte Carlo calculations can involve upward of hundreds of trials using random input numbers and thus could achieve good *precision* in estimating sensitivity with this approach.

Table M.1 Data acquired in individual Monte Carlo trials in which the slope *m* of Fig. P.1 is determined for various assumed values of a particular data point ordinate, y_3

Trial number	y_3	Determined *m*
1	8.1	0.023
2	9.5	0.030
3	8.5	0.025
4	7.5	0.020
5	8.9	0.027
	0.7616	*0.003808*
	-----------Standard deviation-----------	

MPR

Multiplanar reformatting.

MUGA

Multiple-gated acquisition.

Multiplanar reformatting

Creating *slice* views from a 3D *image* with their *planes* having desired orientations. These latter include *axial, coronal, sagittal*, as well as *oblique*. The 3D image consists of information in the form of *voxel* values of *activity concentrations* with coordinates (x, y, z). For an axial slice perpendicular to the *long axis*, that is, z-axis, of the subject, the desired value of z would be fixed. Then the various x and y coordinates would enable selection of voxels that are now *pixels* in the 2D axial slice. In a similar fashion, coronal and sagittal slices may be produced.

Beyond these common orientations, others may be used as well for slices. For example, it is desirable to view cardiac images using the planes in Fig. H.2.

Multiple-gated acquisition

A multi*gated* acquisition scan where frames are triggered, and a form of *radionu-clide imaging* for studying an organ using *planar* or *SPECT* methods. This category of gated scans has come to mean one in which electrocardiogram signals are used for gating a heart scan. Many *frames* are sequentially acquired for subsequent averaging into images at multiple desired times in the cardiac cycle. Acronym is *MUGA*.

Multiple-time graphical analysis

A method of obtaining descriptive *parameters* having physiological significance from plots whose points at various times are computed from *dynamic scan* data and possibly also *tracer* blood sampling. The most common methods here are *Patlak plots* and *Logan plots*. However, other approaches are sometimes used. These typically formulate some type of *model* that permits some form of the *scan* and blood data to be plotted, commonly as a straight line best fitting the data points.

Results of multiple-time graphical analysis are most always a *slope* and *intercept* of a line fitting the data. This type of analysis can be more informative than quantitative markers from a scan based on a single *frame*. However, it tends to be less informative than more complex modeling approaches for data fitting, including *compartmental modeling* with *nonlinear parameter identification*.

Myocardial blood flow

Perfusion for the myocardium. Acronym is *MBF*.

NO

National Electrical Manufacturers Association

A leading trade association in the USA whose members are manufacturers of electroindustry products. One of its useful functions is to provide agreed upon standards for equipment including medical devices. Acronym is *NEMA*.

NEC

Noise equivalent count rate.

NECR

Noise equivalent count rate.

NEMA

National Electrical Manufacturers Association.

Noise

Any part of an information-carrying process that is not the true or original form of the information but is introduced by aspects of the communication (in a general sense) mechanism. Though this latter may be an acoustical device, electronic device, etc., in *imaging*, it would be the *scanner* plus its *reconstruction algorithm*. A common form of noise consists of significant undesirable random fluctuations in *pixel* (*voxel*) values that are superimposed on the ideal true values associated with objects being viewed. Noise interferes with precise determinations of quantifiers.

J.A. Thie, *Nuclear Medicine Imaging: An Encyclopedic Dictionary*,
DOI 10.1007/978-3-642-25035-4_13, © Springer-Verlag Berlin Heidelberg 2012

The commonly encountered noise in images is due to the random nature of the detection process and is visually perceived as graininess. This corresponds to small random *pixel* (*voxel*) variations in value superimposed on a true *mean* value from *uptake*, which can be called the signal. Noise is caused by the randomness in the *radioactive* process as well as by some features of *reconstruction*.

The concept of noise also arises in data analysis. Any sequence of data that should plot as a straight line or smooth curve or line can show somewhat randomly occurring departures from this ideal representation. These departures are of an unwanted nature and are quantified in a *residual*.

Example: In Fig. P.1, the three data points do not fall exactly on the fitted line. There is no physiological reason for this here, and the reason is slight measurement errors. This is referred to as measurement noise.

Noise equivalent count rate

An adjusted *PET scanner's count rate* that results from a specified *activity concentration* within. The coincidence count rate is the sum of true *T*, scattered *S*, and random *R* coincidences. A scattered coincidence involves one of the two *photons* from a disintegration having departed from its original path in transmission to the detector, thereby giving a false *line of response*. The latter also occurs from coincidences just due to chance. The true coincidences are adjusted downward for effects of scatter and random coincidences according to the formula:

$$\frac{T}{1 + S/T + 2R/T}$$

This noise equivalent count rate enables somewhat fair comparisons to be made among *scanners*, with the true count rate being penalized for any substantial scattered and random count rates also present. Besides the specified activity concentration, the use of either a *2D mode* or a *3D mode* substantially influences the result. The largest attainable noise equivalent count rate occurring at an optimal activity concentration for a given mode is one type of scanner specification. More detail in specification would be obtaining the noise equivalent count rate under conditions of various activity concentrations. Acronyms are *NEC* and *NECR*.

Example: A PET scanner in its 2D mode uses a *phantom* having a known 10-kBq/ml activity concentration to measure the NEC for this *concentration*. The values of *T*, *S*, and *R* are measured as 25, 5, and 8 kcps, respectively. The NEC for this 10 kBq/ml is therefore $25 \div [1 + (5/25) + (2 \times 8/25)] = 13.6$ kcps.

Nonlinear parameter identification

A consequence of a mathematical *model* in which some *parameters* do not appear as separate data coefficients to the first power in the equations used to evaluate these from data fitting. Typically, *iterative* guessing is then used to find the set of parameters that best fits the data. See also *kinetic analysis*, *linear parameter identification*, and *parameter identification*.

Example: Fig. P.1 shows a *least squares* fit of three data points to a straight line. An attempt to find a better model than this straight line might assume a series of three equations of the form $y_i = A \times \exp(\alpha x_i)$. These equations have the known x_i and y_i values as well as the unknown parameters A and α. Finding the latter can involve a somewhat complicated process, nonlinear parameter identification. This is because, in contrast to requirements for linear parameter identification, the functional form (i.e., presence of $\exp(\alpha x_i)$ and its being multiplied by A) having the parameters is an impediment to an easy analytical solution.

Normal

When used to describe a *distribution*, a curtailment of *normal distribution*.

Normal distribution

A commonly encountered type of *statistical distribution* that arises when each value comes about by the summed effect of a large number of independent random values. A mathematical consequence of such a process with a *standard deviation* σ is that the *probability density* $= A \times \exp(-(x - x_{avg})^2/2\sigma^2)$, where $A = 1/[(2\pi)^{1/2}\sigma]$. A plot of this probability density is bell-shaped such as depicted in Fig. F.2. Its characteristics include values of a quantity x within ± 1 *standard deviation* σ of the *mean* x_{avg} occurring with a 68% probability and within $\pm 1.96\sigma$ from the mean occurring with a 95% probability. These probabilities are the fractions of the total *AUC* of this probability density function plot for the specified ranges.

Example: The shape of a normal distribution is known to represent reasonably the *distribution* of *FDG-PET SUVs* in Fig. H.1. As described in the probability density example, the calculation of the probability densities for the six midpoints of SUV ranges would give 0.03, 0.27, 0.69, 0.68, 0.28, 0.05. If *least squares* curve-fitting software is given these values, the six bin midpoint SUVs, and the above formula, it can then determine the values of x_{avg} and σ that give the best fit. The result of doing this is $x_{avg} = 2.75$ and $\sigma = 0.52$.

Normalize

To make something conform to a standard or bring about a consistency with respect to a reference. It often consists of dividing individual values in a related set of numbers by some appropriate quantity, quite often having the same units as the values. The purpose is to have normalized results that can be more meaningful, useful, and/or have less undesirable variability. As just one of its useful applications, the individual detectors of *scanners* are adjusted by normalizing factors to account for effects such as their separate *counting efficiencies*, thereby bringing about data consistency for subsequent *reconstruction*. Among other uses encountered in *imaging* are the uses of s*tandardized uptake value* and *tumor-to-normal*. In these, a local *activity concentration* is normalized by the average activity concentration in the entire body or by that in a normal reference tissue respectively.

Example: It is realized that small children and large adults should require different *doses* of injected *tracer* for consistent acceptable *images* from a scanner. Hence, as a simple approach in a certain protocol, an institution decides it is reasonable to always inject 4 MBq for each kg of weight. To adhere to this injection policy in a 70-kg patient, an *injected dose* of $4 \times 70 = 280$ MBq would be used. This patient's normalized dose is $280/70 = 4$ MBq/kg as desired.

Normalized time

The *integrated* plasma *concentration Cp* of a *tracer* divided by a *normalizing* factor, namely, the value of this concentration at the end of the integration time: $\int Cp dt / Cp(t)$. Conceptually, this is an adjusted time *postinjection* that is influenced by the plasma concentration time behavior. A consequence of this definition is the actual mid*frame* time being enhanced by the ratio (average plasma concentration prior to this time)/ (plasma concentration at this time). With $Cp(t)$ diminishing as time increases, the equivalent time is larger than real time. Its principal use is for the abscissa of a *Patlak plot*.

Example: A 2-*exponential* fit to a tracer concentration, normalized to 1 at $t = 0$, that approximates blood samples is $Cp = 0.6\exp(-0.16t) + 0.4\exp(-0.012t)$, with t in min. It is desired to obtain the normalized time at 40 and at 60 min. Evaluating this expression at these times gives $Cp(40) = 0.2485$ and $Cp(60) = 0.1947$. The plasma integrals' values can make use of the formula for the integral of $A \times \exp(-\alpha t)$ being $A \times (1 - \exp(-\alpha t))/\alpha$ between 0 and t: $\int Cp dt$ at 40 min is 16.45 and at 60 min is 20.86. The normalized times, as the quotient of the integral and Cp, are $16.45/0.2485 = 66.2$ min and $20.86/0.1947 = 107.1$ min. Expectedly, these are somewhat longer than the corresponding actual times of 40 and 60 min respectively.

Nucleus

As encountered in nuclear and medical physics, the central part of an *atom*. It consists of a mixture of protons and neutrons bound together and making up virtually all the weight of the atom. The total number of these, referred to as a mass number, is close to the actual atomic weight. This latter is a scale of relative atomic masses where carbon with a mass number of 12 also has an atomic weight of 12. This mass number is the numerical designator used in specifying a particular *isotope* of an atom, such as, for example, F-18.

Nyquist frequency

A *frequency* equal to half the sampling rate used in digitizing a continuously varying process. In *imaging*, a varying process encountered is the sequence of *activity concentration* values in a row of *pixels*. If all frequency content in the actual data being digitized is at and below the Nyquist frequency, it can be unambiguously quantified by the chosen sampling rate. This sampling rate is 1/(sampling increment) with units of cycles per unit time or cycles per unit distance for temporal or spatial information respectively. It provides two or more data values within all repeating behavior intervals having frequencies up to the Nyquist frequency and thus adequately describes these. See also *cutoff frequency* and *resolution*.

Example: If in Table F.1 the *pixel size* is 3 mm, then the sampling increment being used is 3 mm. The sampling rate is (1 cycle)/(3 mm) = 0.333 cycles/mm. The Nyquist frequency is half this, namely, 0.167 cycles/mm. Periodicities for subsequent display in an image at frequencies up to 0.167 cycles/mm are being adequately sampled. However, if there would be some higher frequency content present in the subject, for example, some 0.333 cycles/mm behavior (i.e., repeating patterns every 3 mm), this would result in an ambiguity in the digitized data. The latter would not be able to distinguish it from frequency content below the Nyquist frequency.

Oblique

Slanting or inclined in direction or course or position neither parallel to nor perpendicular to an orientation regarded as conventional. This can describe a *plane* that is not parallel to any of the *coronal*, *transaxial*, and *sagittal planes*. Being at a 45° angle to one or more of these could be an example. Oblique views are convenient for the heart because its *long axis* is not parallel to the body axis.

Overlap

The phenomenon of coinciding partially or wholly; extending over and covering a part of. As applied to *scans* having multiple *bed positions* this is the extent to which the same volume in the subject is scanned twice: once each during each of two successive bed positions. Overlap can be quantified by a percentage of *bed* motion distance between two positions. *Reconstruction* requirements of *2D mode* scans dictate that typically only a couple percent overlap may be sufficient. However, substantially more can be required for *3D mode* reconstructions.

PACS

Picture archiving and communication system used in radiology to manage an encountered multitude of *images* with associated information for their use in varieties of applications of these. The hardware and software of this system accommodate interfaces among acquisition devices, workstations, mass storage devices, and various other user needs.

Parameter

Any factor that defines a system and determines (or limits) its performance. As a special quantifier, such as some constant characteristic of a system, a parameter would appear in a mathematical *model* apart from the latter's continuously varying variables. In model equations, it typically may be an additive term or part of a coefficient of a variable's expression. Values of parameters, such as *rate constants*, can determine how a model responds to input variables.

Example: In a *Patlak plot*, the straight line fit is described by $Q/Cp = Ki \times T + V$. There are two parameters in this plot of tissue *activity concentration Q* divided by plasma *tracer concentration Cp* against *normalized time T*: one is the *slope* of the line as the *influx constant Ki*; the other is the *intercept V*.

Parameter identification

A process of finding *model parameters* that gives a best fit of the model to the data points from a system. Various *algorithms* exist for determining parameters that best meet some fitting criterion. This latter would be some *cost function* that is optimized. In some cases, analytical formulae exist that give parameters in terms of data

J.A. Thie, *Nuclear Medicine Imaging: An Encyclopedic Dictionary*,
DOI 10.1007/978-3-642-25035-4_14, © Springer-Verlag Berlin Heidelberg 2012

being fit. In other cases, *iterative* guesses may be used. See also *kinetic analysis*, *linear parameter identification*, and *nonlinear parameter identification*.

Example: In Fig. P.1, a straight line model is chosen to fit its three data points. The parameters *slope* and *intercept* are identified as 0.025 min^{-1} and 0.5 respectively.

Parametric image

An *image* where, instead of a customary-acquired data display, other computed results are displayed at each *pixel* (*voxel*) in their stead. One such choice for a parametric image can be where each pixel (voxel) is the *influx constant* parameter obtained from *Patlak* analyses of a *dynamic scan* data for that pixel (voxel). One advantage of a parametric image over a usual *activity concentration* image can sometimes be providing better *contrast* between regions, such as pathological versus adjacent normal. This would be due to circumstances in which the chosen parameter is somewhat highly influenced by the pathological character of the tissue – more so than the normally imaged activity concentration.

Example: Normally, as in Table F.2, the pixel values are assumed to come from activity concentrations being measured by the *scanner*. Alternatively, a dynamic scan might have been done in which a separate *Patlak* analysis for each pixel's time behavior would yield an influx constant for that pixel. These values would replace those of Table F.2 in constructing the display of Fig. F.1.

Partial volume effect

The smearing out of a *scanned* object's true *activity concentration* (that should appear at each *pixel* (*voxel*)) into a wider displayed pattern because of the lack of perfect scanner *resolution* for small objects (i.e., having a dimension near or less than the scanner's *full width at half maximum* of its *point spread function*). This occurs because even for an ideal point *source* of activity concentration, the *image* would display less than this value at this object's pixel (voxel) and correspondingly displays additional contributions to values at surrounding pixels (voxels). When partial volume corrections are made, the observed image activity concentrations at pixel (voxel) locations are adjusted by factors that convert these to values which the object actually has at these locations. See also *spillover* and *spill-in*.

Example: In Fig. R.1, it is seen how a bar with a uniform activity concentration appears in an image where the *FWHM* somewhat exceeds the bar width. The 8×4 region of pixels corresponding to just the bar's actual location displays the sum of its 32 pixel values as only 224. This is only part of the bar's actual $32 \times 18 = 576$ total of pixel activity concentrations present. Additionally, the central pixels of the display each shows only half of the 18 actually present.

Partition coefficient

A ratio of *concentrations* of two related forms of a substance in a system. When adapting this concept to *compartments* in a *model*, it is the ratio Q_2/Q_1 of two equilibrium *activity concentrations*. This typically would be when Q_1 and Q_2 are both changing very little with time or otherwise are at least changing at the same percent per unit time. Evidently, the partition coefficient can be one way of characterizing *uptake*. Large values of (Q_2 = tissue activity concentration)/(Q_1 = plasma activity concentration) indicate a substantial ability of this tissue to store *tracer*.

Example: A simple application of the partition coefficient is to obtain the ratio of *rate constants* in instances where a special tissue's only interaction with a plasma tracer is to exchange it through a cell wall in the simplest of models, the one shown in Fig. C.3. When equilibrium is achieved, the forward K_1Cp and reverse k_2Q rates are equal. Here, K_1 and k_2 are *rate constants* for transport into and out of the cell; Cp and Q are plasma and cell concentrations respectively.

$$K_1Cp = k_2Q$$

$$K_1 / k_2 = Q / Cp$$

Hence, a rate constant ratio can be determined by knowing Q from the *image* and Cp from an image blood region or by blood sampling.

Patlak plot

A plot of a tissue-to-plasma *activity concentration* ratio, Q/Cp, as an ordinate against *normalized time* as the abscissa. Under certain often encountered conditions met at later times in a *dynamic scan*, data points corresponding to midtimes of various *frames* can be well approximated by a straight line fit. The *slope* of this line is the *influx constant*. See also *multiple-time graphical analysis*.

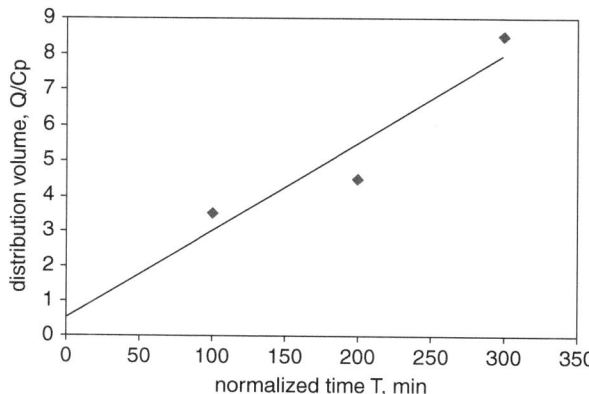

Fig. P.1 Patlak plot example from data points based on measurements of a region's Q and other measurements of Cp corresponding to the same times

Example: Results of fitting a generic straight line, $y = mx + b$, to three data points by a *least squares* fitting *algorithm* are shown in Fig. P.1. The line *slope m* is 0.025 min^{-1} as the influx constant and its *intercept* is 0.5.

Percent injected dose

Indicated as *%ID*, the amount of *activity* present in a region or organ as a percent of total available *injected dose*. The specific calculation is

$$\%ID = 100 \times (\text{activity in a region}) \div (\text{injected dose})$$

Quite commonly, especially for small animals, the region is taken to be a unit mass. Then, rather than total activity, its *specific activity* is used to obtain a related quantity:

$$\%ID / g = 100 \times (\text{activity in 1 g}) \div (\text{injected dose})$$

When the %ID/g is multiplied by (subject weight in grams)/100, the result is the *standardized uptake value* divided by that region's density ρ, that is, SUV/ρ.

Example: A *dose* of 8 kBq of *FDG* is injected into a 20-g mouse for a *PET scan*. The overall body average *concentration* before any excretion is 8/20=0.4 kBq/g. A *hot spot* region of 0.25 g is measured with an average specific activity of 1.2 kBq/g corresponding to 0.25 × 1.2=0.3 kBq present in it. The %ID for this region is 100 × 0.3/8=3.75%. The %ID/g is 100 × 1.2/8=15%/g. This may be converted to the region's SUV/ρ as 15 × 20/100=3. As a check on this, the SUV directly calculated from the ratio of region activity per unit volume to the body average specific activity is (1.2 kBq/g) × ρ/(0.4 kBq/g)=3ρ. For tissues commonly encountered, it is usual to take ρ as 1 g/ml.

Perfusion

The process of a flooding through the arterial and capillary network to saturate the surrounding tissue. In particular, perfusion can quantify a *blood flow* rate density in tissue as the volume of blood per unit time (such as ml/min) passing through a designated mass (such as 100 g) of tissue. Thus, perfusion is a quotient of a blood flow rate and its associated tissue mass. Typical units are ml/100 g/min.

Example: The average perfusion in the brain can be computed from knowledge of the flow rate into the brain and the brain mass. If the former is 756 ml/min in a subject with a brain mass of 1,400 g, the quotient of these is (756 ml/min) ÷ (1,400 g)=0.54 ml/g/min=54 ml/100 g/min

PET

Positron emission tomography.

PET/CT

Hybrid imaging using *PET* and *CT*. These two *imaging* modalities are performed on the subject while remaining on the *bed*. Advantages are: having both structural images and *functional images* with moreover their *fusion* assisting in interpretations and being able to use *attenuation coefficient* information from the CT *scan* in lieu of a separate *transmission scan* for PET for an *attenuation correction*.

Phantom

Imaging phantom.

Pharmacokinetics

The characteristic movements of drugs within biological systems, as affected by absorption, distribution, binding, blocking, elimination, biotransformation, and excretion; particularly the rates of such movements. The understanding of these movements over time is typically formulated in a mathematical *model*. This latter then lends itself to useful numerical applications in the analysis of biological data. A special case of pharmacokinetics is the *compartmental modeling* used to describe *tracer uptake* for purposes of performing *kinetic analysis*.

Phase

A distinguishable part, or a stage, in a series of events or in a process of development. When quantified, it can be a measure of separation of some event from some starting designated time t_o, such as often in a cyclic process. For an event at time t, the phase can be expressed as a time delay, $t - t_o$. In a cyclic process, it can be expressed as a phase angle in degrees of

$$360 \times (t - t_o) / (\text{cycle's period})$$

Example: A *gated scan* is performed in which the electrocardiogram's R wave peak in used to trigger each *frame*, and thus its time is t_o. When a *tracer's uptake* has reached equilibrium, a *voxel* in the myocardium still fluctuates in the *reconstructed activity concentration* as the wall thickness fluctuates throughout the cardiac cycle. It is found that a particular *voxel* shows a peak value at 320 ms after the start of the cycle at t_o. The phase of this peak may be expressed as 320 ms. For a duration of the cardiac cycle of 800 ms, the phase is also $360 \times 320/800 = 144°$.

Phase analysis

Measuring successive *phases* of events in individual cycles in repetitive processes, such as the cardiac cycle, and then determining quantitative markers from this set. This can be done to characterize how cycle-averaged phases behave over many cycles acquired at various conditions and locations. If the phase is constant for every cycle or for every condition at a given location, no phase analysis is possible beyond a *mean* value for phase. But if there is some fluctuation in the data, then additional quantitative analysis is possible. In particular, the *standard deviation* of these fluctuations can be calculated. Also, *parametric images* of the phase at each *pixel* (*voxel*) can be useful.

Example: Cycle-averaged phase data is collected individually for many voxels to study phase behavior in the myocardium. This data, expressed in degrees, consists of many values such as 315, 320, 330, 320, ... Each phase value designates the separation in time of a local *activity concentration* and a reproducible starting point taken from a peak in an electrocardiogram. These phases would be found to have an average value of 320° and a standard deviation of 15° for the series of many values suggested here. Additionally, it is informative to examine the *histogram* of these phases. Pathologies in which the heart exhibits dyssynchronous behavior can be detected by their large standard deviations and anomalous histogram shapes. Quantitative features of the latter can be associated with pathologies.

Photon

A smallest observable single packet of electromagnetic *radiation*, generally considered to be a discrete particle having no mass or charge. In *imaging*, the *gammas* being emitted by a *radioactive* substance are considered to be a stream of photons when they are individually counted by detectors. This photon concept applies to all forms of electromagnetic radiation even though wavelike behavior is also used in characterizing it. An example of this latter is the bending of visible light when it passes from one medium to another different one. Yet the concept of photons as traveling particles also applies.

Pinhole camera

A special *gamma camera* having only one pinhole instead of multiple parallel holes as its *collimator*. While good *resolution* is achieved as the hole is made smaller, there are other considerations involving design compromises: a sufficient *count rate* to avoid *noise* and a suitable subject area which can be encompassed in the *image*. The principle of imaging through a pinhole is a quite ancient one for optical systems.

Pixel

The smallest resolvable rectangular area of an *image*, either on a display or stored in memory. Pixel is a shortened form of the phrase picture element. This smallest element of area (most always a square) in a 2D display has an associated *pixel size*. For a display, a *gray scale* or *color scale* is applied within this area. The entire image then is made up of such areas. It is possible to see individual pixels in the magnified display, Fig. S.2. See also *voxel*.

Pixel size

The distance on the *imaged* subject that corresponds to the width (or the height typically the same as the width) of the smallest piece of the subject that is displayed as a *pixel*. This size depends on selections made using the *reconstruction* software. The user makes decisions as to the number of pixels and their size that he wishes to satisfactorily represent the subject. See also *voxel size*.

Planar imaging

Implementation of a *gamma camera* to obtain 2D *images* with no *tomographic reconstruction* process being involved. Either one view or two *conjugate views* for combining would be obtained. This imaging modality predates the era of *tomography*. It resembles ordinary reflected light photography in the capability of presenting a subject view. However, it is based on *tracer* emissions that occur at various depths in the subject and are transmitted with various *attenuations*.

Plane

An imaginary surface formed by a sweeping rotation of a line through point; a flat surface that can totally contain straight lines between any pair of points on it. A plane can be described by three points in space. Common designations in *imaging* for some planes are *coronal, sagittal, transaxial*, and *oblique*. Within this last category, the three planes used in cardiology are designated according to the axis lying within the plane: *horizontal long axis, vertical long axis*, and *short axis*. See also *slice*.

Point spread function

The displayed values in an *image* that result from an ideal point *source*. This 3D function is generally described by a section cut through it in which the abscissa shows relative distance from the point and the ordinate the *activity concentration*.

This spreading out of the point source is due to the lack of perfect *resolution*. See also *line spread function*, *partial volume effect*, and *spillover*.

Example: A section through the point spread function as measured in a *scanner* by imaging just a very small *radioactive* source within the *field of view* is shown in Fig. F.2. It is typically characterized by its *full width at half maximum* as illustrated.

Poisson distribution

A *distribution function* describing the probabilities of the occurrences of a selected number of independently random events in a chosen time or space domain interval. Additionally, these probabilities apply when the number of occurrences per unit time or space remains constant on average. This special *probability distribution* in particular can apply to the number of independent *radioactive* disintegrations occurring in a given time interval when knowing their average rate of occurrence over a very long interval. A characteristic of this *distribution* is that the *standard deviation* of a Poisson process is expected to be the square root of the average number of events occurring in the given interval.

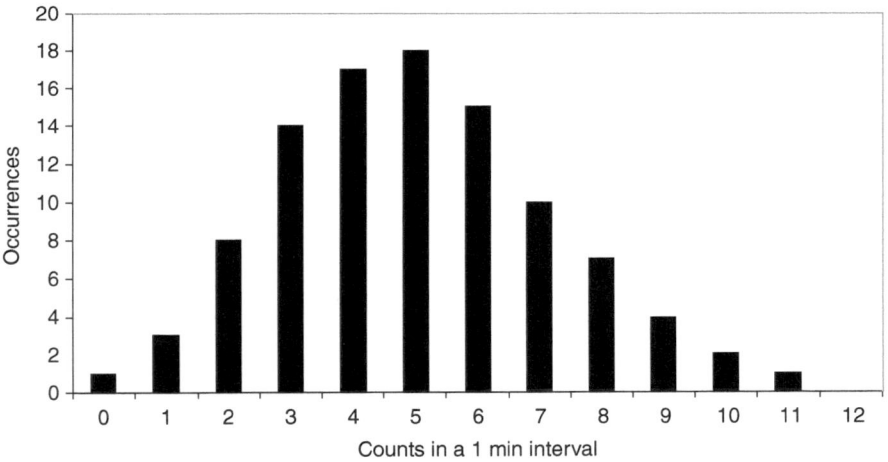

Fig. P.2 Number of counts obtained in a 1-min interval for 100 trials counting emissions of a *radioactive* source whose average *count rate* is 5 cpm during this test

Example: Fig. P.2 shows a *histogram* conforming to the shape of a Poisson distribution expected from counting a very weak radioactive *source*. (Values plotted here may be from statistical software or from a formula.) It is characterized by a *mean* number of counts in the 1-min interval being only 5. The histogram shows that having exactly 5 counts occurs 18 times. Other numbers of counts also occur though not as frequent. It can readily be verified that summing for the histogram bars (number of counts in a 1-min interval) × (number of occurrences of such an event) gives 500. Then, dividing this by the 100 trials results in 5 as the average. Since this is not a large number, some asymmetry can be seen in the histogram. The standard deviation may also be computed from the data of the histogram and is 2.2, which agrees with the expected √5.

Polar map

A 2-dimensional display in which the value plotted, such as by using a *color scale*, is located on the display by its radial coordinate and an angular or azimuthal coordinate. When *gray scale* or *color scale* values are displayed at the polar map's points, these represent averages for local areas. A common special case of a polar map is all points having the same radius. The plot then just uses azimuthal information to locate the plotted values.

A special application of polar maps in *imaging* utilizes concentric annuli to depict any type of myocardial tissue quantifier that is associated with *planes* of the *short axis*. The outermost annulus displays quantifiers corresponding to the *circumferential profile* at the myocardial base. Interior to this, successively smaller annuli represent various annuli of tissue as one progresses toward the apex. A central circle displays the apex quantifier. This type of polar map would result if a *color scale* of quantifiers were the makeup of the wall of a 3D hollow cone structure that approximates the shape of the myocardium and which would be sliced and then crushed along its axis into a 2D display.

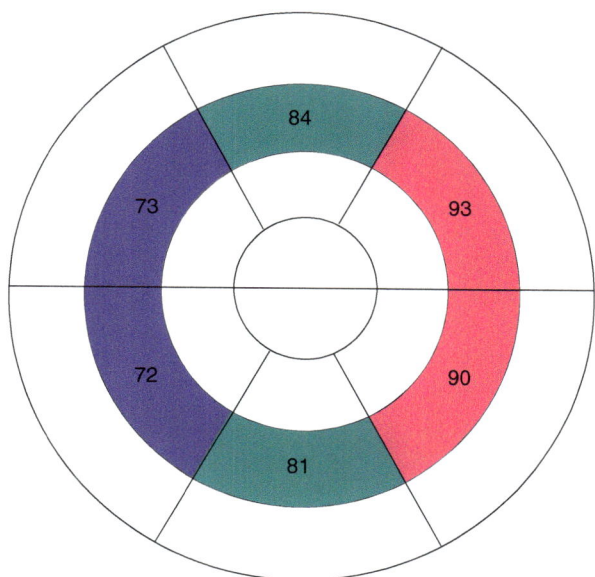

Fig. P.3 Polar map whose *segments* are a 20 *voxel* representation of the myocardial *uptake*, each having an associated quantifier. This map, shown in a process of construction, has slice sectors filled in according to a *color scale* representation of the numerical values (not normally shown as here) associated with the sectors

Example: The displayed segments of one particular myocardial short axis *slice* show numerical values in one of the annuli of Fig. P.3. It is easily verified that these are averages over 60-degree intervals of the circumferential profile of myocardial *activity concentrations* shown in Fig. C.1. Similarly, remaining values in other annuli of this figure could be obtained from circumferential profiles of other slices. When all the sectors are quantified and a *color scale* used, then the plot is referred to as a *bull's eye*.

Positron

Positive *beta* particle. It is the antiparticle of the *electron*, having the same mass but being positively rather than negatively charged. Moreover, unlike the electron, the positron is not a naturally occurring particle. It appears sometimes in disintegrations of *radioisotopes*. But then its existence is short-lived because it collides with an electron found throughout mater. This collision results in mutual *annihilation* and concurrent emission of a pair of 511-keV *photons*.

Example: Some positron emitters used in tracers in *PET* are carbon-11, nitrogen-14, oxygen-15, fluorine-18, and rubidium-82. All but the last are produced in a *cyclotron* which is usually at the PET site or at least nearby because of *half-life* considerations.

Positron emission tomography

An *imaging* technique based on measuring the *photons* produced by collisions of *electrons* and *positrons* within living tissue. In positron emission tomography, a subject is given a *dose* of a positron-emitting *radionuclide* attached to a substance which can interact with a subject's tissues. When living tissue containing the positron emitter has its electrons encountering the latter, photons produced by collisions of electrons and positrons are detected by a *scanner* as shown in Fig. P.4, revealing in fine detail the tissue location of the substance administered. Two photons almost 180° apart emitted for each mutual *annihilation* of a positron and an electron provide an identified *line of response* when coincidentally detected. This provides data for the *reconstruction process* of *computed tomography*. See also *electronic collimation*. Acronym is *PET*.

Posterior

Denoting the back surface of the body; at or near the hind end in quadrupeds or toward the spine in primates (as opposed to *anterior*).

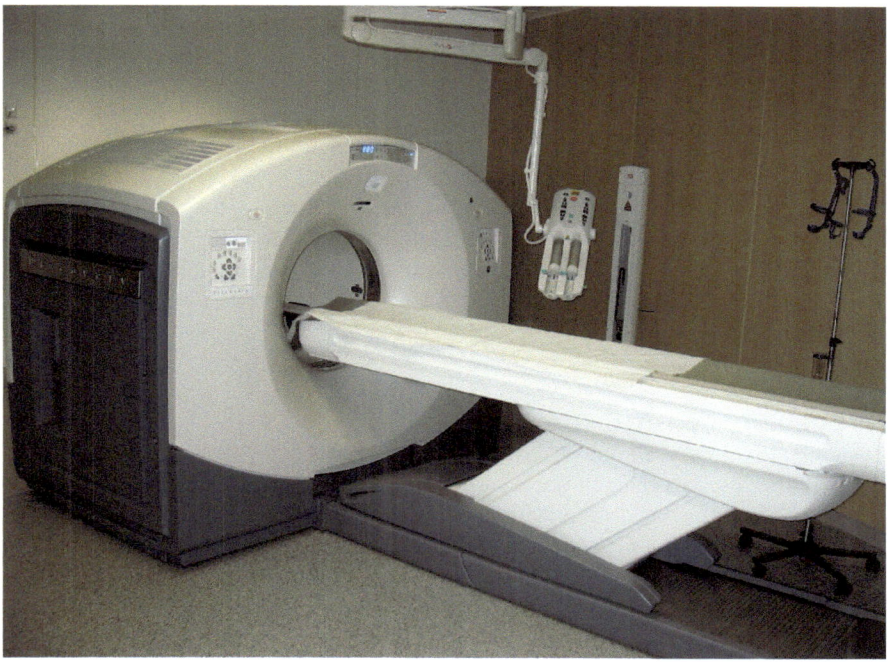

Fig. P.4 *PET/CT* showing the *gantry* housing the detectors (the *left center*) and the moveable *bed* (the *right foreground*). As the bed moves the patient into the gantry interior a portion of his body is scanned, the *axial* length of which is the *field of view* located within the gantry. In the *whole body scan*, the bed pauses at successive positions while sections are scanned. Both the PET and the *CT scans* can take place while the patient remains on the bed (Reprinted with permission from the Wikimedia Commons repository of the Wikimedia Foundation from file, 16slicePETCT.jpg, http://commons.wikimedia.org/wiki/. Accessed 28 September 2011)

Postinjection

Pertaining to the time period starting when *tracer* injection for a *scan* is initiated. *Uptake* takes place during this period. For purposes of calculations in *dynamic scans*, it is convenient to assign $t = 0$ when injection starts.

Precision

A quantitative representation of the degree of an *accuracy* component necessary for or associated with a particular measuring action. Precision is one component of the overall *accuracy* of a result. If there is no source of *bias* from the methodology, instrument, etc., then the precision and accuracy are the same. It characterizes the *reproducibility* of a measurement in a number of independent trials under similar conditions. *Standard deviation*, *standard error*, and *coefficient of variation* are common statistical measures of precision. Also, a simple measure might also be the difference of the highest and lowest value in a reproducibility study or this difference expressed as a fraction or percent of the *mean*.

Example: Successive *SUV* results for the same tissue in a patient in an older *PET* scanner, not recently calibrated, are: 2.3, 2.8, 3.2, 2.0, 2.4, 2.7, 1.8, 3.6, 2.6, and 2.4. The precision is the standard deviation of these, namely, 0.54. This represents a $0.54 \div 2.6 = 0.21$ or 21% coefficient of variation for this *mean* SUV of 2.6. However, this is not the accuracy of the result because there can additionally be a bias from systematic error due to slow drifts over time of the scanner's *calibration factor* since its last calibration.

Probability density

A quantifier used to characterize a *statistical distribution*. It describes the probability of a variable having a value within a small unit band around this value. It can also be determined from a *histogram* each of whose bars contain the number of occurrences within the bin width at a particular value. The probability associated with occurrences in this bin is its number of occurrences divided by the total number in all bins. The probability density then is this resulting probability divided by the bin width. It has the units of probability per unit value.

Example: The same organ's *SUVs* are determined in *FDG-PET scans* for 200 patients having similar pathology, with results in Table H.1 plotted in Fig. H.1. From this data, it is possible to determine the probability densities that correspond to the various bins. Each number of occurrences in Table H.1 is divided by 200 and again by the 0.5 bin width. Thus for these three occurrences near 1.5, the probability density is $(3 \div 200) \div 0.5 = 0.03$ per SUV unit. Such test data may then be used to assess likelihoods of certain results in future studies of this tissue. Thus with this low probability density SUV, values near 1.5 would be regarded as uncommon. Also a useful result from this data can be a *least squares* fit of the 6 probability densities to a formula, as shown in the *normal distribution* example.

Probability distribution

Statistical distribution.

Projection

Detector data acquired in a specified direction from the subject. It represents a view from a certain direction. The concept may refer to one or more *lines of response* as well as entire *images*. In a 2D projection image, each *pixel* represents a characterization of *activity concentrations* along a viewing line through the subject. These might be the average of activity concentrations. However, in a *maximum intensity projection*, only the largest activity concentration along the viewing line would characterize it.

When a *gamma camera* acquires an *image*, it is in a certain position relative to the subject. This would be referred to as a projection with an associated modifier describing the direction. Designations such as *lateral* view and lateral projection are synonymous.

Prone

An *anterior* recumbent body position whereby the subject lies on the stomach and faces downward (as opposed to *supine*).

Proximal

Situated nearest to a point of attachment or origin (as opposed to *distal*).

p-value

A measure of the probability that a result happened by chance. The lower the p-value, the more likely it is that the result was caused by some phenomenon of interest. It is used in association with a result having some random uncertainty being compared to a hypothesized value or circumstance. The p-value then is the probability that the observed difference could have come about by chance, notwithstanding any intrinsic reasons that this difference should be a real effect. When *p* is small, such as below an almost universally used 0.05, the result is said to be *statistically significant*.

Example: The *normal distribution* and *probability density* examples show that probability densities computed from the *histogram* of Fig. H.1 are represented by $[\exp(-(x-x_{avg})^2/2\sigma^2)]/[(2\pi)^{1/2}\sigma]$. *Least squares* fitting of this expression to this data results in x_{avg} being an *SUV* value of 2.75 and *standard deviation* $\sigma = 0.52$. A property of normal distributions is that values more than 1.96 standard deviations in either direction from the x_{avg}, including both above and below it, occur only 0.05 of the time. Hence the p-value for encountering new subjects having SUVs below $2.75 - 1.96 \times 0.52 = 1.73$ or above $2.75 + 1.96 \times 0.52 = 3.77$ is 0.05. This probability is low enough that such patients could be classified as abnormal, recognizing, however, some small uncertainty in making this judgment.

QA

Quality assurance.

QC

Quality control.

Quality assurance

Programs of regular assessment of facilities and activities to evaluate and ensure that criteria, standards, and procedures are adhered to and that delivered products or services meet performance requirements. This program encompasses all measures taken to verify that the best performance is being obtained from both equipment and procedures. Aspects of *quality control* can appear in a broad quality assurance program, though sometimes the terms quality control and quality assurance are loosely used interchangeably. Acronym is *QA*.

Quality control

Set of measurements and inspections taken to verify that performance of equipment and procedures remains within specified limits. These commonly consist of various appropriate checks conducted periodically at times outside of normal equipment use. They are specially designed to detect departures from its ability to perform normal functions satisfactorily. Sometimes the terms *quality assurance* and quality control are loosely used interchangeably. Acronym is *QC*.

J.A. Thie, *Nuclear Medicine Imaging: An Encyclopedic Dictionary*,
DOI 10.1007/978-3-642-25035-4_15, © Springer-Verlag Berlin Heidelberg 2012

Example: Varieties of quality control tests are performed on *SPECT scanners*. Some common tests are:

Various calibrations
Uniform cylindrical *phantom scan*, including a *sensitivity* measurement
Comparing mechanical axis of rotation with centers of projected *images*
Resolutions in a phantom having a variety of object sizes

Quality factor

A factor assigned to a type of *ionizing radiation* in converting *absorbed dose* measured in *grays* to a biologically *equivalent dose* measured in *sieverts*. In formula form, (equivalent dose) = (quality factor) × (absorbed dose). This factor is exactly 1 for 200-keV x-rays. It is however taken as 1 for other *energies* of x-rays, *photons, electrons,* and *positrons*. Other types of *radiation* can be more damaging to tissue, according to some selected criterion and for a given absorbed dose, than those having a quality factor of 1. These are assigned higher values, and thus it requires less absorbed dose of these to cause the same biological consequences as the same dose of x-rays, photons, electrons, or positrons. Other terms for the quality factor are *relative biological effectiveness* and radiation weighting factor.

Quantitation

The act of measuring or estimating a quantity. In *imaging*, this involves the obtaining of useful numerical results from a *tracer's uptake*, such as in specific regions. Quantitation is supplementary to *visual interpretation* in diagnostic imaging. Numerous methodologies are in use for performing quantitation. Some are rather simple to implement, such as *scoring*; others can be much more complex such as *nonlinear parameter identification* in *models*. Fortunately, in the era of highly developed user-friendly computer software, special mathematical skills are not always required for implementation of a number of popular quantitation tools. See also *semiquantitative* and *visual interpretation*.

R

Roentgen.

Rad

A unit for *absorbed dose* equal to the amount of *energy* from any type of *ionizing radiation* (e.g., alpha, *beta*, *photons*, neutrons, etc.) deposited in any medium (e.g., water, tissue, air). A *dose* of 1 rad means the absorption of 100 ergs per gram of absorbing tissue (100 rad = 1 Gy). The term is the commonly used contraction of *radiation absorbed dose*. This energy density value is a purely physical characterization of the *radiation* received without regard to biological effects. The number of rads of radiation becomes more meaningful when its effects on living tissue are considered. Hence, there is a process of converting the number of rads to what is meaningful for living tissue, taking into account the type of tissue and type of radiation. See also *equivalent dose, quality factor*, and *sieverts*.

Radiation

Emission or propagation of electromagnetic *energy* (waves/rays), or the waves/rays themselves, a stream of fundamental particles (*electrons*, neutrons, protons, alpha particles) or a mixture of these. In *nuclear* and *atomic* physics, these types of energy are released from changes of state within atoms or nuclei or from subatomic particle kinetics. Depending on its effect on the matter through which it passes, it may be *ionizing radiation* or nonionizing radiation. In *imaging*, the types of radiation in the form of electromagnetic waves encountered are x-rays and *photons*. See also *radioactive* and *radioactivity*.

J.A. Thie, *Nuclear Medicine Imaging: An Encyclopedic Dictionary*,
DOI 10.1007/978-3-642-25035-4_16, © Springer-Verlag Berlin Heidelberg 2012

Radiation absorbed dose

Rad.

Radioactive

The characterization of a substance having *radioactivity*. Thus, it would not include x-ray devices. However, a substance giving off various particles or giving off *gamma* rays, similar in nature to x-rays, would be called radioactive.

Radioactive source

The substance which is *radioactive*. A common usage of this term is also to designate a sealed radioactive *source* consisting of typically one *radioisotope* in a small quantity. Popular uses of sealed sources include equipment calibrations.

Radioactivity

The quality of emitting or the emission of corpuscular or electromagnetic *radiations* consequent to *nuclear* disintegration, this being a natural property of all chemical elements of *atomic* number above 83 and possible by being induced in other elements. In *imaging*, the common form of radioactivity encountered are *gamma* rays. The latter come from a *radionuclide* in a *tracer*. See also *radioactive*.

Radioisotope

A version of a chemical element that has an unstable *nucleus* and emits *radiation* during its *decay* to a stable form. A chemical element may have a number of *isotopes*. But it is those which emit radiation that are radioisotopes.

Radionuclide

Radioisotope.

Radionuclide imaging

Scintigraphy.

Radiopharmaceutical

Substance having a *radioisotope* and normally intended for some type of ingestion or introduction into a living organism for medical or biological reasons. In *imaging*, a radiopharmaceutical would be used as a *tracer*, such as the popular *FDG* in *PET*.

Rate constant

Parameter appearing in *models* to describe a unidirectional transfer rate out of a *compartment*. It is the (amount transferred per unit time) ÷ (amount present in the compartment) and usually designated by the symbol k. This would be the fraction transferred per unit time if the numerator and denominator amounts are specified with same units, as quite usually the case. When designated as k_i, the i is a digit assigned to the specific transfer process. It is usual to first formulate a *compartmental model* describing a process. Then the quantifiers in this model are principally the rate constants associated with transfers.

Example: Tissue data of a *PET* neurotransmitter *dynamic scan* study is analyzed using a compartmental model. For the first compartment, which is *tracer* in plasma, the amount present is designated as Cp with units of µBq/ml. The amount transferred from plasma by a unidirectional process into a tissue per unit time is traditionally designated as $K_1 Cp$ (rather than $k_1 Cp$). Also it is given somewhat customary units of µBq/(g of tissue)/min. In a particular instance of *nonlinear parameter identification*, K_1 is found to have a value of 0.1 ml/(g of tissue)/min. The product $K_1 Cp$ then would mean, for example, if $Cp = 10$ µBq/ml were present in plasma that $0.1 \times 10 = 1$ µBq/(g of tissue)/min is a unidirectional transfer rate into tissue.

RBE

Relative biological effectiveness; quality factor.

Rebinning

Sorting *image* acquisition data into specially chosen classes or bins which differ from those pertaining to the original acquisition. A common type of rebinning is processing *list mode* data in order to achieve specially designated *frames*. Then a bin would correspond to a desired time duration around a *mean* frame time. Data meeting this criterion is then segregated into bins, which are frames, each of which then undergoes *reconstruction*.

Receptor

A protein located on the cell surface, or in the cytoplasm, that binds to a specific signaling factor, such as a hormone, antigen, or neurotransmitter, causing a conformational and functional change in the receptor molecule. A *ligand*-bound receptor then alters its interaction with other molecules, which leads to changes in cellular physiology through modification of the activity of one or more signal transduction pathways. A number of *imaging* applications take advantage of having a *tracer* ligand being imaged in this binding process. *Compartmental modeling* of this is used to obtain quantifiers from *scan* data.

Reconstruction

The process of generating an *image* from the raw detector data, or set of unprocessed measurements, made by an imaging system. Input information consists of detected counts associated with the *lines of response* within the subject. One of a variety of *algorithms* is used to transform this data, to make appropriate corrections, and eventually to arrive at an image giving locations and magnitudes of these individual *sources* of *activity concentrations* in the subject for the displayed image. See also *sinogram*.

Rectilinear scan

A very simplified *scan*, now of historical interest, in which a *radiation* detector is systematically positioned over the subject, viewing only a very small region at a time. The detector is repositioned along a desired scan line as it sequentially collects data. The latter is recorded for these positions along scan lines and stored for an eventual display of all these small regions. Scans of parallel lines when shown together can give a 2D *image* display. These scans are a forerunner of *planar imaging* which acquires data from substantial volumes of the subject at the same time.

Reference region

A *region of interest* in an *image* chosen for comparison purposes because its *uptake* properties have some desired feature. Thus, in a *tumor-to-normal* ratio, the reference region could be an appropriate nontumor tissue that may serve this purpose of *normalization*. Similarly, in neuroimaging, it is common to use the cerebellum or a region contralateral to the region of interest as a reference region in calculating ratios of *activity concentrations*.

Example: In *visual interpretation*, the reader often qualitatively compares the image intensity of a particular region with that of another region. The latter may be surrounding tissue, a contralateral region, or an organ such as the liver. These are regarded as being somewhat of a standard. An intrinsic reason for this could be relatively low variability in their *SUVs* in a population. Sometimes, a *score* is assigned to quantify this comparison to a reference region. But for more *precision*, a quantifier with continuous values is (*ROI's* activity concentration) ÷ (reference region's activity concentration).

Region of interest

A user-selected area within a 2D *image*. The choice is guided by knowledge that *activity concentrations* for the *pixels* within the boundary *contour* of this region will be used in quantifying its particular feature. A number of contiguous pixels are enclosed by manual selection or by a computer *algorithm*. Popular for the latter are pixels with activity concentrations that exceed a threshold percentage of the region's *maximum pixel* and are within a boundary contour line that results. When manual regions of interest are drawn on 2D images by a reader, these can be circles, ellipses, and even free-form boundaries that enclose contiguous pixels. See also *volume of interest*. Acronym is *ROI*.

Example: A *hot spot* is visually identified in an image, a portion of whose pixel values are shown in Fig. C.4. The pixels of this hot spot are segregated by a drawn *contour* shown, thus creating a region of interest. This ROI is characterized by the average activity concentration within it, that is, for all 8 pixels within this oval. It can be verified that this average is 5.5 here.

Registration

Two *images* (as from the same *scanner* at different times or from different scanners) of the same anatomical region in a subject being positioned relative to each other so their individual *pixel* (*voxel*) locations best correspond to each other according to specified criteria. A common use for registration arises in obtaining *fused images*. If there is no fusion, a *CT* or MRI anatomical image and another scanner image based on *uptake* could only be viewed side by side, with the reader's mental processes providing organ location coordination between these. However, with the implementation of a registration *algorithm*, it is possible to achieve a best possible matching of pixels (voxels) used in a fused image.

A number of considerations arise in registration. *Pixel* (*voxel*) *sizes* must be the same. Angular orientations of the subject along axes must correspond, as must dimensions of organs in various directions. Adjustments (rotating, rescaling, and warping) are made in the images so that impartial criteria for a satisfactory matching are met.

Relative biological effectiveness

Quality factor.

Rem

Roentgen equivalent man.

Reorientation

Presentation of *image* views other than the standard *coronal*, *sagittal*, and *transaxial* views. These three standard views are all mutually at right angles to each other. But occasions can arise where other orientations are more convenient to view. These are then termed *oblique*.

Example: The most common circumstance for requiring oblique views arises in cardiac imaging. Since natural axes in describing heart geometry do not coincide with axes associated with the three standard views, reorientation is performed. The resulting oblique views shown in the reorientation of Fig. H.2 are then quite convenient for reading.

Reproducibility

A quantified extent to which a number of measurement results expected to be nearly the same in fact vary somewhat from each other. Average of differences occurring in a number of pairs of same-subject test and retest results is one simple method of assessing reproducibility. Also, simply the *standard deviation* of a set of results of a quantity not otherwise expected to change much could be another. See also *precision*.

Example: A *scanner* is used to monitor effects of chemotherapy with monthly scans of the lesion being treated. Results are *SUVs*. But the question arises as to the minimum detectable change in SUV that can reliably be used in interpreting treatment changes. To determine this, a similar lesion is scanned a number of times. For this reproducibility data, the patient repetitively undergoes these scans within a few days time when the lesion *activity concentration* would be virtually unchanged. Successive SUV values are 4.9, 4.6, 5.2, 5.4, 6.1, 6.0, 3.5, 4.9, 5.3, and 4.4. From these, a 0.77 *standard deviation* can be computed and taken as an indication of reproducibility. This suggests that most SUV results are within about 0.77 of their likely true value. Hence, in monitoring chemotherapy over long periods of time, it would only be changes in SUV a reasonably significant amount beyond this 0.77 that would be examined for possible physiological significance.

Residual

Remaining or left behind. In data analysis, it has come to mean some measure of the difference between a calculated result and a data. For an individual point, this might be the actual difference of these or its absolute value, or this difference squared. For multiple data points, the sum of the squares of these differences is often employed as a residual.

Example. An *algorithm* for *least squares* fitting of the straight line of Fig. P.1 to data can involve computing residuals for various values of the *parameters m* and *b*. This residual is the sum of the squares of the fitting errors,

$$\left(y_1 - mx_1 - b\right)^2 + \left(y_2 - mx_2 - b\right)^2 + \left(y_3 - mx_3 - b\right)^2$$

In Fig. P.1, the (x_i, y_i) points are (100, 3.5), (200, 4.5), and (300, 8.5). Five pairs of *m* and *b* values may be tried: (0.024, 0.5), (0.025, 0.5), (0.026, 0.5), (0.025, 0.4), and (0.025, 0.6). The residuals for these five trials are 1.64, 1.5, 1.64, 1.53, and 1.53, respectively. The set of parameters giving the best fit is when the residual minimizes at 1.5, namely, $m = 0.025$ and $b = 0.5$. In practice, when an *iterative* approach is used, it can take numerous guesses to find a minimum residual.

Reslicing

Changing from one prescribed method of obtaining 2D *slices* from a 3D *image* to another. This other method may have a different thickness and/or direction of cut through the subject than the original set of slices. Slicing so as to have certain *oblique* views can be convenient for the reader.

Resolution

The size of the smallest element that can be separated from neighboring elements. In an *image*, viewing of details below a resolution distance is highly impaired if not impossible. A popular measure of *scanner* resolution is the *full width at half maximum* of the *point spread function*. A practical measure of visual resolution is the largest number of *line pairs* per unit length that can be distinguished as individual lines. In describing resolution, attributes such as "high," "good," etc., correspond to readily discernible smaller sizes, lower *FWHMs*, and higher line pairs per unit length. See also *cutoff frequency*.

In digital imaging, an important factor in resolution is the *pixel size d*. A set of alternating black and white columns 1 *pixel* wide will have each line pair occupying a distance $2d$. The maximum number of line pairs per unit length that can be readily resolved is $1/2d$ if there are no other *filtering* effects present.

R

A concept of resolution can also be encountered in other dimensions. Temporal resolution would be characterized by the smallest time increment capability available to separate events. *Energy* resolution is described by the *full width at half maximum* of the energy *distribution* for the type of *radiation* as detected by imaging instrumentation. Being able to select the center of this distribution and limit the width with good resolution enables a detector to be quite selective to a particular type of radiation in the presence of radiation at other energies.

0	0	0	0	0	0	0	0	0	0	0	0	0
0	0	0	0	0	0	0	0	0	0	0	0	0
0	0	0	0	0	0	0	0	0	0	0	0	0
0	0	0	0	0	0	0	0	0	0	0	0	0
0	0	0	0	18	18	18	18	0	0	0	0	0
0	0	0	0	18	18	18	18	0	0	0	0	0
0	0	0	0	18	18	18	18	0	0	0	0	0
0	0	0	0	18	18	18	18	0	0	0	0	0
0	0	0	0	18	18	18	18	0	0	0	0	0
0	0	0	0	18	18	18	18	0	0	0	0	0
0	0	0	0	18	18	18	18	0	0	0	0	0
0	0	0	0	18	18	18	18	0	0	0	0	0
0	0	0	0	0	0	0	0	0	0	0	0	0
0	0	0	0	0	0	0	0	0	0	0	0	0
0	0	0	0	0	0	0	0	0	0	0	0	0
0	0	0	0	0	0	0	0	0	0	0	0	0

0	0	0	1	1	1	1	1	1	1	0	0	0
0	0	1	1	1	2	2	1	1	1	0	0	
0	1	1	2	2	3	3	2	2	1	1	0	
1	1	2	3	4	4	4	4	3	2	1	1	
1	2	3	4	5	6	6	5	4	3	2	1	
1	2	3	5	6	7	7	6	5	3	2	1	
1	2	4	6	7	8	8	7	6	4	2	1	
1	2	4	6	8	9	9	8	6	4	2	1	
1	2	4	6	8	9	9	8	6	4	2	1	
1	2	4	6	7	8	8	7	6	4	2	1	
1	2	3	5	6	7	7	6	5	3	2	1	
1	2	3	4	5	6	6	5	4	3	2	1	
1	1	2	3	4	4	4	4	3	2	1	1	
0	1	1	2	2	3	3	2	2	1	1	0	
0	0	1	1	1	2	2	1	1	1	0	0	
0	0	0	1	1	1	1	1	1	0	0	0	

Fig. R.1 Detail with (1 mm × 1 mm) *pixel* values that would result in a *slice* through a 4-mm-thick and 8-mm-wide bar *phantom* whose length is perpendicular to this view. The *plane* of the slice is parallel to end faces of this long bar and perpendicular to the bar's *long axis*. On the left are actual *activity concentrations* in the bar and surrounding *background* as if it were displayed perfectly. On the right are image results from having a 6-mm FWHM scanner resolution

Example: The bar image pixel values on the right in Fig. R.1 have been numerically computed from its uniform activity concentration as affected by a *scanner's point spread function*. The latter has the form shown in Fig. F.2, though with a FWHM = 6 mm. Edge smearing caused by the filter width is seen to be substantial in the image. This is because the FWHM somewhat exceeds the bar thickness of 4 mm. These indistinct boundaries would make it somewhat difficult to discern the bar from another parallel one (not shown) if the latter would be close.

Robust

A desirable characteristic of a method in which its results would be rather unaffected by certain conditions under which these were obtained. The results are said to be robust with respect to these potentially influencing conditions in contrast to other methods where changeable conditions can lead to changeable results.

Example: An institution with a new *scanner* checks its *activity concentration* calibration result using a standard *phantom* filled with a known prepared uniform activity concentration. Additionally, it compares the activity concentration result in a normal liver of the first patient of the day against the published population averages of such values elsewhere. Of these two methods, in spite of the clinical appeal of the second, the first is more robust. This is because, regardless of which might have the greater *precision*, the phantom has the advantage of being a *reproducible* standard. A single patient's result could be susceptible to off-normal liver conditions not known to the technologists.

Roentgen

A unit of exposure to ionizing *radiation*. One roentgen is the amount of *photons* or x-rays required to produce ions resulting in a charge of 2.58×10^{-4} C/kg of dry air at 1 atm pressure and 0°C. Since 33.97 J of *energy* are known to be associated with an ion pair having 1 C of charge, the product $(0.000258 \text{ C/kg}) \times (33.97 \text{ J/C}) = 0.00876$ J/kg which characterizes *energy* deposition of 1 R in air. With the *gray* and *rad* being 1 and 0.01 J/kg, respectively, this means 0.00876 Gy and 0.876 rad of *absorbed dose* is due to 1 R in air. The roentgen is a historical unit of exposure used for x-rays and *gammas*. Abbreviation is *R*.

Roentgen equivalent man

Commonly called *rem*, a standard unit that measures the effects of *ionizing radiation* on humans. The *equivalent dose* in rems is equal to the *absorbed dose* in *rads* multiplied by the *quality factor* for the type of radiation. It is also possible additionally to make effectiveness adjustments for the distributions of the subject's radiation exposure among various tissues for which its relative effects differ. An alternative unit is 1 Sv = 100 rem.

ROI

Region of interest.

Sagittal

Pertaining to a *plane* containing a line parallel to the *long axis* of the subject's body and additionally giving a left or right view. This plane is perpendicular to both the *transaxial* and *coronal* planes. An example of a sagittal view is Fig. F.3. See also Fig. A.2.

Scan

The *image* or its data obtained by gathering viewing information with a sensing device. The specific type of data acquisition for a scan involves the separate detections from the many parts of the subject and subsequent assembling into an image. This contrasts with image production by radiosensitive surface techniques such as radiography and *autoradiography*.

Scintigraphy

An *imaging* technique that uses a small *dose* of a *radioactive* chemical called a *tracer* that enters and spreads through a subject for purposes of its emissions being detected by a *gamma camera* with its imaging system. Common usage tends to apply this term more to *planar imaging* than to *nuclear tomographic* modalities. Yet usage sometimes extends to any *gamma camera* modality. See also *autoradiography*.

Scintillation detector

A *sensitive* crystal that converts *ionizing radiation* to flashes of light which in turn are sensed by an optically coupled photomultiplier converting these to electrical pulses. The latter have a proportionality to the *energy* of the *radiation*, thereby permitting a useful feature of using electronics to select a particular energy band of radiation of interest.

Scintillation detectors are used to detect *photons* in *planar imaging*, *SPECT*, and *PET*. Key to their success is having developed crystal materials with advantageous properties of *sensitivity* along with capabilities of detecting large numbers of events per unit time.

Score

A number or range of numeric values measuring performance, function, quality, or ability. In characterizing degrees of severity, as of a region in an *image*, a special scale of scores can be devised by a reader to assist his *visual interpretation*. A scoring scale could have low numbers representing near normal and high numbers highly diseased. Sometimes, symbols, such as – and +, are used in lieu of numbers.

Table S.1 A scoring system sometimes used in visual interpretation of images

	Score
Definitely normal	1
Probably normal	2
Equivocal	3
Probably diseased	4
Definitely diseased	5

Example: In his visual interpreting of a *PET scan,* a reader notes the relative brightness and other diagnostic indicators of a selected tissue region. After making a judgment based on experience with similar cases, he scores in accordance with ad hoc rules he has implicitly adopted when classifying into the categories of Table S.1.

Scout scan

Topogram.

SD

Standard deviation.

SE

Standard error.

Segmentation

Partitioning an *image* into two or more differing regions with separating boundaries based on desired characteristics within these as defined by their *pixel* (*voxel*) values. A motive is to facilitate subsequent analyses that will use these portions of the image containing the more appropriate information desired for the study.

Image analysis software can be conveniently used in segmentation. In each of one or more steps, it is possible to start with all pixels (voxels) within a selected region and specify rules regarding which of these regions are kept for the next step and which are discarded. A typical step might involve keeping only those having *activity concentration* values between certain upper and lower limits. See also *contour*.

SEM

Standard error of the mean which is synonymous with *standard error*.

Semiquantitative

As colloquially used, a designation for a simpler *quantitative* method that contrasts with a more rigorous one used for a similar purpose. Often, the terminology, semiquantitative analysis, is used in *imaging* as a synonym for usage of the *standardized uptake value*. This is in contrast with any more extensive analysis approach such as a *Patlak* plot or *nonlinear parameter identification* in a *model*.

Sensitivity

1. The ability to respond to physical stimuli or to register small physical amounts or differences. This can be a measure of the minimum change in an input signal that an instrument can detect. Also a *normalized* sensitivity would be an observed change detected divided by some standardized value of input causing it. Thus, a measurement of sensitivity could use a known *activity concentration* in an unattenuated *source* introduced within a *scanner* and measure some change in detector *count rate*. Inversely related to this concept of scanner sensitivity is its *calibration factor* for a volumetrically distributed uniform activity concentration: this latter divided by the corresponding displayed uniform count rate per *voxel* in its *image*.
2. The fraction of all the positive/abnormal cases that are diagnosed correctly when a certain methodology is applied to all the positive or abnormal cases. This is calculated by (number of correct positive or abnormal diagnoses) ÷ (total number of positive or abnormal cases). This measure is useful in comparing effectiveness of diagnostic methodologies in positive/abnormal populations. See also *accuracy*.

Septa

Parallel *photon* absorbing plates close to detectors that restrict *PET* photon reception from all directions from the *scanned* subject except in a somewhat narrow *slice* perpendicular to the subject's axis. Septa are present in a *2D mode* but are retracted in a *3D mode*.

Short axis

Line through and perpendicular to an object's *long axis*. This line may intersect the long axis anywhere within the object.

Colloquially in cardiology, this refers to a plane which is a *short-axis* view, seen in Fig. H.2, and contains the short axis. A number of parallel planes would define *slices* whose *images* show the enhanced *uptake* of near-circular annular myocardial wall sections. These can provide data for *circumferential profiles* which can then make up a *bull's eye* display.

Sievert

The International System (SI) unit for *equivalent dose* of *radiation* equal to 1 J/kg. 1 Sv = 100 rem. The equivalence is one of having the same biological effect for the particular living tissue and type of radiation. Thus the sievert takes into account biological considerations beyond merely physical *energy* deposition.

Unlike the *gray* which can be directly measured by an instrument, sieverts must be calculated from grays for the particular radiation and its distribution over the body. Thus if more than one type of radiation is present, concurrently or sequentially, the number of sieverts would be calculated for each and the result summed to give the total equivalent dose from all. Additionally this equivalent dose may often be converted to an effective *dose* for the entire body by using weighting factors in calculations which take into account how the radiation is distributed and differently affects the various tissues and organs. Thus radiation to the gonads would receive more weight than that to other body tissues. Abbreviation is Sv. See also *ionizing radiation*.

Example: In a particular *PET/CT scan*, 15 mGy is received by a patient during his or her *CT* scan. Then, the effect of the *FDG* tracer results in an additional 7 mGy on average received by body tissues. With a *quality factor* of 1 for both these radiations, the equivalent dose is $(15 \times 1) + (7 \times 1) = 22$ mSv.

Signal to noise ratio

(Some measure of useful information from a system) ÷ (some measure of interfering unwanted, often random, information also present). In one *imaging* application of this concept, these quantities would be a fixed known *activity concentration* and the *standard deviation* of its inherently fluctuating measured values attributable to the imaging protocol. Acronyms are *S/N* and *SNR*.

Significant

Statistically significant.

Simulation

A technique which attempts to provide an abstract *model* of a particular system. It can utilize a mathematical model, which attempts to predict the behavior of the system from a set of *parameters* and initial conditions given the model. Quite usually, a computer is involved and the simulation is one form of *computer modeling.*

Single-photon emission computed tomography

A type of *tomography* in which *gamma*-emitting *radionuclides* are administered to patients and then detected by one or more *gamma cameras* rotated around the patient. From the series of two-dimensional *images* produced by a *scanner* of the type shown in Fig. S.1, a three-dimensional image can be created by a computer. In obtaining the two-dimensional images, *collimators* define the *lines of response* for the scanner's *gamma* detectors, and then these directions and *count rates* are used in the process of *reconstruction* in a *computed tomography* process. Acronym is *SPECT.*

Single-photon emission tomography

A curtailment of *single-photon emission computed tomography.* Acronym is *SPET.*

Sinogram

A *gray scale* display of detector counts for various *lines of response.* The latter are located by the abscissa being their distance from the central horizontal axis of the *scanner* and their ordinate being their angle ($0°$–$180°$) relative to vertical. The shade of gray at each *pixel* in the sinogram corresponds to the counts for that line of response. The name originates from an off-axis point source resulting in a sinusoidal curve in the display. Sinograms like the one in Fig. S.2 give a convenient view of the detector data acquired for further processing in *image reconstruction.* Their displays can be useful in scanner *quality control.*

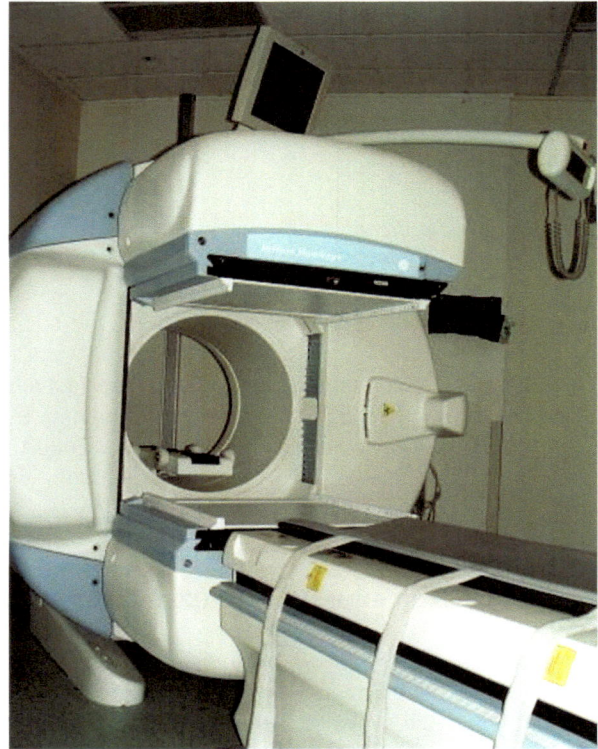

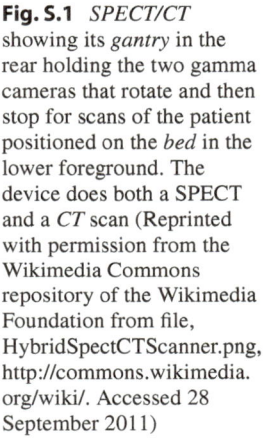

Fig. S.1 *SPECT/CT* showing its *gantry* in the rear holding the two gamma cameras that rotate and then stop for scans of the patient positioned on the *bed* in the lower foreground. The device does both a SPECT and a *CT* scan (Reprinted with permission from the Wikimedia Commons repository of the Wikimedia Foundation from file, HybridSpectCTScanner.png, http://commons.wikimedia. org/wiki/. Accessed 28 September 2011)

Slice

A thin flat piece cut off of some object; anything resembling such a cut off piece. In *imaging,* the 2D display of a slice corresponds to *voxels* between a pair of parallel *planes,* separated by the slice thickness, cutting through the 3D image at a desired location and orientation. The value of each *pixel* is the average of voxels along lines perpendicular to the planes. See also *reslicing.*

Slope

The property possessed by a line or surface that represents the extent of its departure from the horizontal. This is the tangent of the angle it forms with the positive x-axis. It represents the change in the vertically plotted variable (ordinate) per unit of change in the abscissa variable. If (x_1, y_1) and (x_2, y_2) are coordinates of two points on a line, then the slope and tangent of the line's angle with the horizontal is $(y_2 - y_1)/(x_2 - x_1)$.

Example: In Fig. P.1, the slope of the drawn line may be computed from the coordinates of its endpoints, (0 min, 0.5) and (300 min, 8), as $(8 - 0.5)/(300 - 0) = 0.025$ min^{-1}.

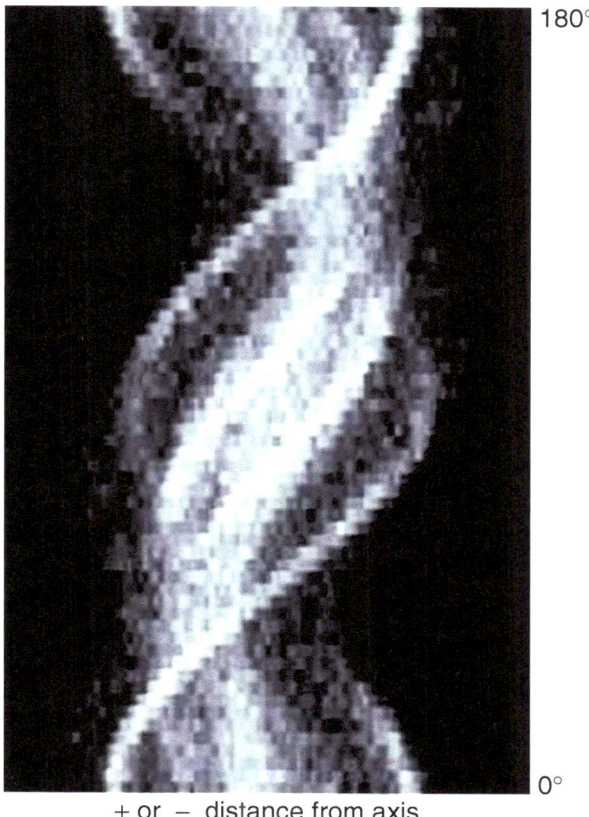

180°

0°

+ or − distance from axis

Fig. S.2 Sinogram from a *SPECT* scan of a *phantom* that includes among other things two off-center *hot spots*. As the angle of viewing increases (from *bottom* to *top* of figure), these appear, when viewed by detectors, at different distances (horizontal in this figure) from the centerline. With this progression of the viewing angle through 180°, the hot spots each trace a sine-wave (the two outermost spirals) from bottom to top of the sinogram. Other off-axis regions of *activity concentration* closer to the axis are also seen here. Also it is noticeable: how a limited number of discrete quantitative values from reconstruction are displayed by a gray scale within square pixels; and how the original display software provides fuzzy edges for these in its chosen resolution. (Reprinted with permission from the Wikimedia Commons repository of the Wikimedia Foundation from file, Spect_sinogram_360.jpg, http://commons.wikimedia.org/wiki/. Accessed 28 September 2011)

Smoothing

The process by which some complexity or detail of an entity is simplified by some type of manipulation. For *imaging*, a common smoothing process is using a spatial *filter* to change the larger *pixel*-to-pixel (or *voxel*-to-voxel) variations in value into more gradual variations spread over somewhat larger distances. Such a filter removes the higher spatial *frequencies*. Thus an image which would have an excessive overall appearance of speckled graininess could be changed to having a more eye-pleasing uniformity in shades of gray. However, edges of regions, previously well defined by large changes in pixel (voxel) values over a range of just a couple pixels (voxels), would appear somewhat fuzzy.

S/N

Signal to noise ratio.

SNR

Signal to noise ratio.

Sokoloff model

A widely used mathematical *model* for *tracer uptake* in *PET*. Originally developed for the brain, it describes inter*compartmental* transports of glucose or its tracers in varieties of tissues to which it has been adapted. These transports involve a plasma compartment, an intermediate compartment having the same glucose form as in plasma, and a metabolic compartment having another molecular state, namely, glucose-6-phosphate. See also *fluorodeoxyglucose*.

Solid-state detector

A sensor of *radiation* in which a semiconductor material is made conductive by the impinging radiation. The resulting electrical pulses from this small volume can then be used for purposes of *imaging*. Additionally this type of detection allows discrimination of *energies* to give assurances of viewing only one desired form of radiation from the subject. Good *sensitivities* along with high *count rate* capabilities have been achieved with special semiconductors.

Source

Radioactive source.

Specific activity

A *quantitative* indicator of the *radioactive* emissions per unit time per some standard unit of measure for the amount of material having this radioactivity. The latter would typically be the total quantity in grams or kilograms for the radioactive plus nonradioactive components of a substance. Alternative units of measure such as volume in ml or *moles* can also be used. Specific activity can be calculated by dividing the number of *becquerels* or *curies* by the number of standard units of measure. Resulting units can be Bq/g and Ci/g. But when volumetric measures are used, the units would be Bq/ml and Ci/ml and the result more customarily be referred to as *activity concentration*. See also *concentration*.

Specific volume

Volume contained in a unit mass. This is the reciprocal of the commonly encountered density, the mass within a unit volume. Its determination would consist of dividing a known volume by its mass. Typical units can be ml/g or l/kg. See also *distribution volume*.

SPECT

Single-photon emission computed tomography.

SPECT/CT

Hybrid imaging using *SPECT* and *CT*. These two imaging modalities are performed on the subject while remaining on the *bed*. Advantages are: having both structural and *functional* images with moreover their *fusion* assisting in interpretations and being able to use *attenuation coefficient* information from the *CT scan* for an *attenuation correction*.

SPET

Single-photon emission tomography; single-photon emission computed tomography.

Spicular

Spikelike aspect of a structure within an *image*. In *visual interpretation* of lesions, the reader can use this characteristic in describing shape.

Spill-in

Phenomenon in a *reconstructed image* where true *activity concentration* of the tissue immediately adjacent to an object being studied appears spatially partially smeared into *pixels* (*voxels*) of this object. Correspondingly, the true activity concentrations in these surroundings are not displayed totally in their own *pixels* (*voxels*). Thus the object's displayed activity concentration is a mixture of its own and that from its environment. See also *partial volume effect, point spread function,* and *spillover.*

Spillover

Phenomenon in a *reconstructed image* where true *activity concentration* of an object is not displayed totally in its corresponding *pixels* (*voxels*). Instead it is spatially partially smeared into nearby pixels (voxels) corresponding to its surrounding medium. See also *partial volume effect, point spread function,* and *spill-in.*

Example: Fig. R.1 shows a uniform activity concentration bar where all pixels would have a value of 18 if it were *imaged* perfectly. The actual image resulting from a *scanner* having a *FWHM* exceeding the bar thickness is also shown. It can be seen that the displayed activity concentration within the bar region is never higher than only 9. However the pixels in the region surrounding the bar do not show a 0 value but instead have values up to 6 due to spillover.

SPM

Statistical parameter mapping.

Standard deviation

A measure of the variability within a range of values for a set of numbers. Standard deviation is a statistic used as a measure of the dispersion or variation in a *distribution* and is equal to the square root of the arithmetic *mean* of the squares of the deviations from the arithmetic mean of the set of values. It is the square root of the *variance* and widely used to characterize uncertainty when stating a measurement result. Generally a correction is made on this result to remove a theoretical *bias* if a limited number n of values are available for its determination for a very large population. The correction is to increase this defined standard deviation by the square root of $n/(n-1)$. Acronym is *SD*.

Example: *SUVs* are obtained in a series of 10 patients all with a lesion having about the same pathology. These are 4.7, 4.3, 5.2, 5.4, 6.2, 6.6, 3.4, 4.8, 5.3, and 4.1. The *mean* SUV here is 5.0. The uncorrected variance is $[(-0.3)^2+(-0.7)^2+(0.2)^2+(0.4)^2+(1.2)^2+(1.6)^2+(-1.6)^2+(-0.2)^2+(0.3)^2+(-0.9)^2]/10=0.828$. Hence an uncorrected standard deviation is $\sqrt{0.828}=0.910$. If corrected for the *bias* stemming from having only 10 patients, the result is $0.910 \times \sqrt{(10/9)}=0.959$.

Standard error

Result of dividing the *standard deviation* by the square root of the total number of cases in a *distribution*. This quotient, (standard deviation) ÷ √n, represents the statistical *precision* of a *mean* of a distribution when this mean is obtained from a set of n similar quantities being averaged. Thus the more values in the set, the more precisely its mean relative to the true mean can be calculated. For *normal distributions,* there is a 68% probability that the measured mean will be within 1 standard error of the true mean. Acronyms are *SE* and *SEM* for the synonymous standard error and *standard error of the mean,* respectively.

Example: The standard deviation was found to be 0.959 in the example given for standard deviation of *SUVs* in 10 patients. This is an indication of the fluctuation in SUV values from patient to patient within this group. For any individual patient's measured SUV, it has a precision of 0.959. The standard error for this group of 10 patients is $0.959/\sqrt{10} = 0.303$. This is a measure of the uncertainty in the group average SUV of 5.0. But if 100 patients had been used in this study, the standard deviation would still be expected to be about 0.959. However the average SUV of these 100 would now be more confidently known, having a standard error of only about $0.959/\sqrt{100} = 0.0959$. If the *statistical distribution* of these SUVs is near *Gaussian,* then the meaning of the 10 or 100 patient result is that there is about a 68% probability of the true SUV falling within a band: $5.0 - 0.303 = 4.7$ to $5.0 + 0.303 = 5.3$ when there are 10 patients and $5 - 0.0959 = 4.9$ to $5 + 0.0959 = 5.1$ when there are 100 patients.

Standard error of the mean

Standard error.

Standardized uptake ratio

A term sometimes historically used for the *standardized uptake value*. Acronym is *SUR.*

Standardized uptake value

A measure of regional *tracer uptake* calculated as [*activity concentration* within a 2D region of interest (ROI) or 3D volume of interest (VOI) measured on a properly calibrated *PET* or *SPECT image* (kBq/ml)]/[*injected dose* (kBq)/body weight (g)]. This results in a g/ml dimension. Thus it is a *normalized* measure of tissue activity concentration. Since the denominator here is the average *specific activity* in the entire body before any excretion, the standardized uptake value is a local to body average ratio. Without any qualifier, it would be understood to be an average *pixel* (*voxel*) value within the defined region. Qualifiers of maximum or peak are used to indicate usage of a region's largest pixel activity concentration or an average for a few pixels that include this largest respectively: SUV_{max} or SUV_{peak}.

While the entire body weight is normally used, in the case of widely employed glucose *tracers,* there is sometimes recognition that these are poorly taken up in fat tissue. Hence, for such tracers, a preferred substitute for body weight might be the lean body mass or some other appropriate function of body *parameters*. The dimensions of the standardized uptake value would normally be g/ml or kg/l. Even if no dimensions are given, these would be understood to be applicable. Acronym is *SUV*. See also *percent injected dose.*

Example: After a 1-h *scan*, the average activity concentration in a *region of interest* is 30 kBq/ml. This 70-kg patient was injected with 370 MBq. The SUV is (30 kBq/ml)/(370,000 kBq/70,000 g)=5.68 g/ml.

Statistical distribution

A representation (often a graph or plot) showing the likelihood that a particular event will occur over a set of events with associated values. The representation may be defined by a mathematical function, the *probability density* function. A use in diagnostic *imaging* can be characterizing how uptakes in a particular tissue in population occur over some range of values. See also *histogram.*

Statistical parameter mapping

Converting throughout a region the *pixels' (voxels') activity concentrations* to a difference from a reference and then *normalized* by a statistical factor. The latter is chosen by statistical theory and software so that a *parametric image* displaying this would emphasize voxels that are *statistically significant*. A subject's Q pixel (voxel) value would be converted to

$$(Q - Q_{ref}) / (\text{a statistical factor})$$

This technique is popular for the brain where an off-normal and reference condition are compared. Thus quite large absolute magnitudes of this quantifier in a *parametric image* of a subject can suggest subregions that are statistically unlikely and therefore classified as off-normal. Acronym is *SPM*.

Statistically significant

Feature from a mathematical measure used to ascertain how convincing is a difference between groups. This difference is said to be statistically significant if it is somewhat greater than what might be expected to happen by chance alone. This term is applied to differences, correlations, cause-and-effect relationships, etc., to indicate that they are noteworthy, unlikely attributable to chance and therefore indicating a systematic effect. In statistics, significant (or highly significant) ordinarily indicates a probability of a real, rather than chance, effect being not less than 95 (or 99) percent. This concept is used in diagnostic *imaging* as a basis to assist in deciding between normal and abnormal. See also *p-value*.

Steady state

Condition of a system, having undergone earlier changes with time, where it has eventually reached an essentially stable unchanging condition. When *tracers* are injected, the initial effect in the subject is a tracer transport by the blood to organs for *uptake* where *activity concentrations* build up and often then decrease as well for some time. It is possible however that eventually, for all practical purposes, there will be an almost unchanging (after *decay* correction to injection time) activity concentration in locations being studied. These then would be said to have achieved steady state, also referred to as an equilibrium condition. At this time, it can be convenient to acquire a somewhat unique *image* when, as counts build up in detectors, there are no effects of changes in the organ that could significantly interfere with the study.

The time chosen for *whole body scans* and single scans of a region tend to be chosen if possible when a somewhat near steady state condition has been reached. In contrast to this, *dynamic scans* are performed while uptakes are changing.

Stereotatic

The precise positioning aspect of a medical procedure, with all three dimensions being involved. Coordinates of features determined in an *image* would be utilized in stereotatic procedures such as certain types of biopsies, *radiation* therapies, and surgeries. Stereotatic procedures can be assisted by imaging when the opacity of the subject prevents availability of adequate visual information during the procedure except for that from the image.

Stroke volume

The difference in a cardiac ventricle's blood capacity taken at times of minimum and maximum blood content. This is *end diastolic volume* less *end systolic volume*. See also *blood flow*, *ejection fraction*, and *volume curve*.

Example: In Fig. V.1, a fully filled ventricle having 120 ml reduces to a minimum 50 ml size. The stroke volume is $120 - 50 = 70$ ml.

Superior

In anatomy indicating higher than a given reference point (as opposed to *inferior*).

Supine

A *posterior* recumbent body position whereby the subject lies on its back and faces upward (as opposed to *prone*).

SUR

Standardized uptake ratio.

Survey meter

A portable detector *sensitive* to *radiation* passing through its thin walls and specifically used to quantify the radiation in an environment to assure personnel safety. By measuring the *dose rate* in an area, it is possible to plan allowable times that personnel may safely remain there.

SUV

Standardized uptake value.

SUV_max

The maximum *standardized uptake value* among the *pixels* (*voxels*) within a *region of interest*. See also *maximum pixel* and *maximum voxel*.

SUV_{peak}

Standardized uptake value of the average for just a few *pixels* (*voxels*) that includes the pixel (voxel) having SUV_{max}. The method of selecting this limited number would be specified as well. Thus it could be pixels (voxels) within a 1-cm-diameter *contour* where the largest *SUVs* appear. It can be preferred to SUV_{max} when the slightly better precision from averaging several pixels is desired.

T

TAC

Time activity curve.

Tag

Label.

Talairach space

A widely accepted standard coordinate system of brain physiologically based regions, that is, an atlas space, to which an individual brain geometry from a *scan* can be transformed and realigned for purposes of matching corresponding regions among brains. Each point in the individual brain is given Talairach coordinates, (x, y, z) for its location in Talairach space. With the wide variations in individual brain size, shape, and structure, being able to transform region locations into a standard template facilitates comparisons of scans among individuals. See also *Broadmann's area.*

Target

An object fixed as a goal or point of some process; also something to point at. A *radiation* target is that which receives the effect of a beam of radiation. This may be a material used in the preparation of a *tracer* and is to be made *radioactive* in a *cyclotron* bombarding it with ions. It may also be a region within a subject that is to receive therapeutic radiation.

J.A. Thie, *Nuclear Medicine Imaging: An Encyclopedic Dictionary,*
DOI 10.1007/978-3-642-25035-4_18, © Springer-Verlag Berlin Heidelberg 2012

Throughput

The number of *scans* performed in some unit of time.

TID

Transient ischemic dilation.

TIFF

A bitmap graphics file format utilizing *tagged* fields. This acronym represents Tagged *Image* File Format. This format used for storing images in a computer would have a suffix, tif, for its files. Like the *JPEG* format, there is a motive of using less computer storage space than an original image file, yet preserving fidelity. Unlike JPEG files, TIFF files can be reedited without any loss of fidelity.

Time activity curve

Plot of *activity concentration* as the ordinate versus time as the abscissa. Data typically would come from a *region of interest* or *volume of interest* from a *dynamic scan* or from blood activity concentration sampling at various times. Acronym is *TAC.*

Time of flight

A method used in *PET scanners* that incorporates travel times of the *positron decay photons* to the detectors in *reconstruction* in order to better localize the positron on the *line of response.* Because of electronic limitations in measuring small times, an upper and lower limit is associated with the measured travel times. Nevertheless, incorporating this additional localization information in *reconstruction* improves the *signal to noise ratio* of the *image*, that is, less graininess attributable to random counts. Acronym is *TOF.*

T/N

Tumor-to-normal.

TOF

Time of flight.

Tomogram

An *image* obtained by *tomography*. This image, made up of many parallel *slices* through the subject, contrasts with a single traditional 2D display, such as an x-ray radiograph. See also *topogram*.

Tomography

Imaging by sections or sectioning. 3D imaging here is a composite of adjoining *slices*, each of which may be viewed separately or otherwise utilized.

Topogram

A 2D *projected image* from a *tomographic* device that does not utilize its full capability of *reconstructing* into *slices*. It can be simply producing 2D x-ray radiographs or *planar images* often for the intention of using these as *scout scans* prior to subsequent tomographic imaging. See also *tomogram*.

Tracer

A substance that is identifiable by virtue of some unique signature, its color, or other distinguishing physical property, such as a *radioactive isotope*, a dye, or inert chemical, that is introduced into a biological or other system and can be followed through the course of a process, providing information on the pattern of events in the process or on the redistribution of the parts, elements, or events involved. For *scanners*, the tracer is a radioactive compound that is introduced in small quantities into a subject's blood for purposes of studying a subject's physiological processes when *imaged*. Each tracer is uniquely radiochemically designed with a specific biologic behavior that best suits motives for its use. It often mimics the behavior of a naturally occurring substance in the subject. See also *label*.

Transaxial

Across (i.e., perpendicular to) the *axial* direction. When describing the *plane* of an *image*, it indicates the plane perpendicular to the *long axis* of the subject's body. This plane is perpendicular to both the *coronal* and *sagittal* planes as in Fig. A.2. See also *transverse plane*.

Transfer constant

Rate constant.

Transient ischemic dilation

(Left ventricular cavity volume during stress) ÷ (left ventricular cavity volume at rest). These volumes can be determined from the *image* of a *tracer* in the blood filling this heart chamber, using *voxel size* and number of voxels within cavity walls. Acronym is *TID*.

Transmission scan

Obtaining *scanner* data for use in making *attenuation corrections*. This consists of measurements with external *source* positions involving *attenuating* paths through the subject. It does not involve subject emission *radioactivity* being detected. This approach to obtaining attenuation correction data is an alternative to using *CT* information. See also *emission scan*.

Transverse plane

An imaginary surface perpendicular to the *long axis* of a subject. In *imaging* this describes the *transaxial* view or *plane* in Fig. A.2.

Tumor-to-normal

A common *normalization* of a tumor *activity concentration,* namely, (tumor activity concentration) ÷ (normal tissue activity concentration). The latter can be chosen as a contralateral region or a nearby tissue or *background* region. Popularity of this quantifier stems from a *robust* nature due to both tissues being imaged together in the same subject. See also *contrast*. Acronym is *T/N*.

Uptake

The absorption by a tissue of some substance, food material, mineral, etc., and its permanent or temporary retention. In *imaging* this normally refers to the passage of the *tracer* from plasma into tissue.

Variance

A measure of the variability in a sample or population. It is calculated as the *mean squared deviation* of n individual values from their common mean. In calculations the divisor n for averaging to obtain a mean is commonly used for a large population variance and the divisor $n - 1$ for a corrected variance from a limited size sample. In a large population with n values of x_i, it is the average of the square of departures from the population mean x_{avg}, thus measuring variability:

$$\Sigma(x_i - x_{avg})^2/n \text{ or } \Sigma(x_i - x_{avg})^2/(n-1)$$

The latter form removes *bias* in estimating variance using a limited size data sample of x_i's taken from a population. The variance is the square of the *standard deviation*.

Example: As in the standard deviation example, *SUVs* are obtained on a series of 10 patients in a region having about the same pathology on each. These are 4.7, 4.3, 5.2, 5.4, 6.2, 6.6, 3.4, 4.8, 5.3, and 4.1. The mean SUV here is 5.0. The variance is $[(-0.3)^2+(-0.7)^2+(0.2)^2+(0.4)^2+(1.2)^2+(1.6)^2+(-1.6)^2+(-0.2)^2+(0.3)^2+(-0.9)^2]/10=0.828$. After removing bias, the final result for the corrected variance is $0.828 \times (10/9)=0.920$.

J.A. Thie, *Nuclear Medicine Imaging: An Encyclopedic Dictionary*,
DOI 10.1007/978-3-642-25035-4_19, © Springer-Verlag Berlin Heidelberg 2012

Ventilation-to-perfusion ratio

(*Activity concentration* of a *tracer* measuring lung air flow per unit volume for a region) ÷ (activity concentration of a tracer measuring lung *blood flow* per unit volume for this region). It is useful for the region here to be an individual *pixel* (*voxel*); then this ratio may be displayed as a *parametric image*. See also *perfusion*. Acronym is *V/Q*.

Ventral

Pertaining to the underside or lower surface of the body (as opposed to *dorsal*).

Vertical long axis

An *oblique plane* through the heart containing its *long axis* and showing only two chambers. This and any vertical plane parallel to it can be called a vertical long axis view. These *slices* are also perpendicular to *horizontal long axis* views as well as *short axis* views as shown in Fig. H.2.

Visual interpretation

Results of perusal of an *image* for information that can be gleaned from the relative intensities that display *tracer uptake* as well as from various other image features.

VOI

Volume of interest.

Volume curve

Plot of a ventricle volume as the ordinate versus time as the abscissa in a cardiac cycle. It would be obtained from volumes determined at particular times in the cycle in a *gated scan*. The maximum and minimum are the *end diastolic volume* and *end systolic volume*, respectively. The values of the *slopes* along this curve are volume velocities, that is, how fast in ml/s the volume is changing. It can also be called the time-volume curve. See also *ejection fraction* and *stroke volume*.

Example: Built-in software in a *SPECT* study automatically determines the surface boundary of the left ventricle and then determines the numbers of *voxels* that give the blood interior volume. In Fig. V.1, the total volume is separately calculated for each *gate* interval.

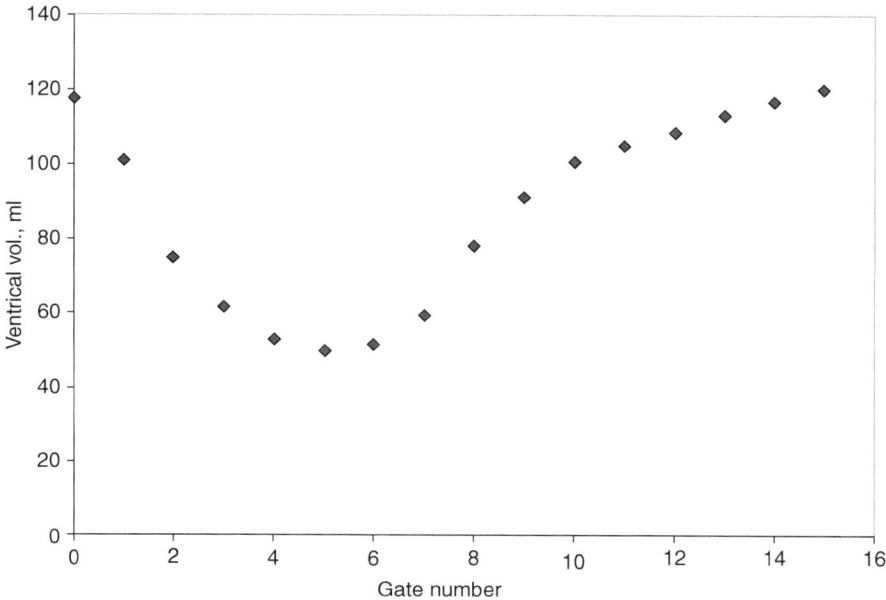

Fig. V.1 A left ventricle volume curve from a gated SPECT study

Volume of distribution

Distribution volume.

Volume of interest

A user-selected volume within a 3D *image*. The choice is guided by knowledge that *activity concentrations* of the *voxels* within the boundary *contour* of this region will be used in quantifying it. A number of contiguous voxels can be enclosed by manual selection or by a computer *algorithm*. Popular for the latter are voxels with activity concentrations that exceed a threshold percentage of the region's *maximum voxel* and are within a boundary *contour* surface that results. See also *region of interest*. Acronym is *VOI*.

Volume rendering

A 2D display of a 3D *image* using one of a variety of *algorithms* that achieve a display of otherwise hidden *voxel* values. The latter would not necessarily be visible in a display due to intervening opacities in the subject that has a range of voxel values. See also *cine* and *maximum intensity projection*.

Voxel

The smallest distinguishable rectangular-parallelepiped-shaped part of a three-dimensional space or image; a shortened form of the phrase volume element. It is the smallest volume element in a 3D display to which a value is assigned. Normally it would have square faces on two bounding *transaxial planes* and have equal rectangular faces for the other four. A *gray scale* or *color scale* can be uniformly applied within this volume for a display. The entire *image* then is made up of such volumes. A voxel's volume is (transaxial plane *pixel* area)×(thickness of *slice*).

Voxel size

The three distances on the *imaged* subject that correspond to the width, height, and depth of the smallest piece of the subject that is displayed as a *voxel*. This size depends on selections made using the *reconstruction* software. The user makes decisions as to the number of voxels and their size that he wishes to use to satisfactorily represent the subject. See also *pixel size*.

V/Q

Ventilation to perfusion ratio.

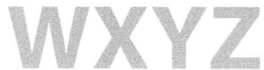

Washout

Used synonymously with *clearance*, the process of a *tracer* leaving a tissue over time. It can be *quantified* by the *clearance rate*.

Well counter

Radiation detector, usually cylindrical, that can accurately quantify the *activity* in a sample placed in a cavity within by registering the individual counts of its emanating radiation. A common form is a hollowed-out crystal based on the principle of detecting its light scintillations induced by the radiation. A use associated with *scanners* is determining the number of *becquerels* of a *tracer* that is to be subsequently injected. See also *dose calibrator*.

Whole body scan

A series of *scans* of a subject taken at sequential *bed positions* as the *bed* moves through the scanner. The *images*, each limited by an *axial field of view*, can then be pieced together to give an extended length image of the subject. A whole body scan as shown in Fig. W.1 contrasts with a single bed position scan in which only a rather limited region within the subject is to be studied.

Fig. W.1 *Coronal* view of an *FDG* whole body *PET* scan. The software has seamlessly joined the images acquired at several bed positions. The brighter areas represent the higher *activity concentrations*. One of these is seen to be the brain whose high *metabolic rate* has resulted in *tracer* accumulation at the time of its *frame*. Substantial tracer in the areas of the heart and bladder is also evident (Reprinted with permission from the Wikimedia Commons repository of the Wikimedia Foundation from file, PET scan image.jpg, http://commons.wikimedia.org/wiki/. Accessed 28 September 2011)

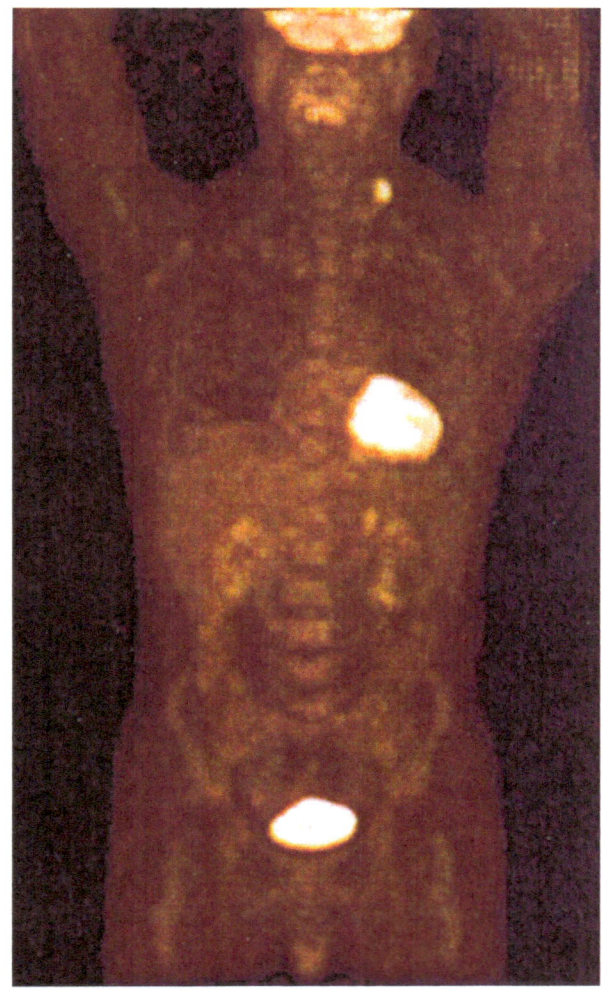

Window

A time, spatial, *energy*, or other type of interval during which something may be achieved, obtained, or observed. One type of interval can be selected upper and lower limits of *activity concentration* in an *image* that then would display only subject features that are within these limits, as when performing *segmentation*. Another type, an energy window, designates a range of *radiation* energies being detected in the neighborhood of a unique energy from the imaged subject. In all instances, the window width is the difference between the upper and lower limits. The window width can also be expressed as a percentage of a principal value within the window. See also *dynamic range*.

Zoom

The factor by which an *image* is expanded in its display when compared to its normal presentation in an original *matrix*. Thus in a *transaxial* view of n pixels in a row or column, the original image has *pixel size* which is (design *field of view* width in the *transaxial plane*)/n. Zooming is achieved by reducing this size by a zoom factor z. The zoomed pixel size is (design *field of view* width in the *transaxial plane*)/$(n \times z)$. In a zoomed display only a portion of the available image is presented, but details can be easier to view.

Accuracy

Precision and accuracy are not the same uncertainty measures if there is a *bias* consideration in addition to random effects. When there also can be bias relative to a true value obtained by another means, then an all-inclusive accuracy term should be used rather than precision.

Activity

When used alone, activity should normally indicate a quantity of *radioactivity* which would be measured in *becquerels* or *curies*. The term, *activity concentration*, rather than a curtailment, activity, is preferable to activity when a *concentration* is being described.

Asymmetry index

Usage of asymmetry index should be accompanied by (a) the particular formula used to calculate it; and (b) any additional description of its terms if needed, such as designations of right and left. Moreover, there can be a need to indicate whether a numerical result is a fraction or a percent. In fractional form, if signed differences rather than absolute values are used, the formulae in use for comparing x_1 and x_2 values are:

$$(x_2 - x_1) / (\tfrac{1}{2}[x_2 + x_1])$$

$$(x_2 - x_1) / (x_2 + x_1)$$

$$(x_2 - x_1) / (\text{either } x_2 \text{ or } x_1)$$

$$x_2 / x_1$$

J.A. Thie, *Nuclear Medicine Imaging: An Encyclopedic Dictionary*,
DOI 10.1007/978-3-642-25035-4, © Springer-Verlag Berlin Heidelberg 2012

Blood flow

If used when the concept of *perfusion* is intended, it would indicate a flow rate density and have typical dimensions, ml/100 g/min. Otherwise, usage of blood flow is to indicate the concept of a volume blood flow rate passing a specified location and have typical dimensions, ml/s.

Blood volume

It should be made clear, if not obvious from the context, whether blood volume is its volume (in liters) in the subject, a dimensionless fractional volume in a region, or the blood volume per unit of tissue amount in a region.

Contrast

If a number is given for contrast between two regions quantified by a larger Q_2 and smaller Q_1, the formula being used for its computation should be known: Q_2/Q_1 for the contrast ratio; $(Q_2 - Q_1)/Q_1$ for the fraction; and $(Q_2 - Q_1)/(Q_2 + Q_1)$ for the normalized difference.

DAR

See the commonly preferred synonym, *standardized uptake value*.

Differential absorption ratio

See the commonly preferred synonym, *standardized uptake value*.

Differential uptake ratio

See the commonly preferred synonym, *standardized uptake value*.

Distribution activity ratio

See the commonly preferred synonym, *standardized uptake value*.

Dose

It can be appropriate to indicate whether this is: (a) an administered dose (such as an amount of *activity*); (b) *absorbed dose*; or (c) *equivalent dose*. Giving units will distinguish the first from the latter two.

Dose rate

It can be appropriate to indicate whether this rate is associated with: (a) an administered dose (such as an amount of *activity*); (b) *absorbed dose*; or (c) *equivalent dose* when the term is used apart from its context or is not clear from its units.

DUR

See the commonly preferred synonym, *standardized uptake value*.

Gamma

While often used colloquially as synonymous with photon, gammas are a special type of the more encompassing term, photons. Unique to gammas is their origin in a *decaying* nucleus. Thus in the *positron* and *electron annihilation* occurring in *PET*, it is appropriate to indicate that *photons*, rather than *gammas*, result.

Glucose level

Stating this as glucose blood level, glucose plasma level, or glucose serum level is appropriate when specific details of the method of measurement are not given. Typically glucose *concentration* in plasma and serum is ~11% and ~16% higher, respectively, than in whole blood.

Half-life

If the context in which half-life is used is not clear, then there can sometimes be uncertainty as to the type of half-life involved. In *nuclear* medicine, the overwhelming usage is that of the physical half-life associated only with the *radioactive decay* process. However, on some occasions it can be appropriate to be more specific when concepts of *biological half-life* or *effective half-life* are involved.

Horizontal long axis

This description of an *image* display here is a curtailment of the more rigorous phrase, horizontal long axis view.

Log

Good practice is subscripting log with a descriptor delineating whether it is a common or natural *logarithm*, i.e., $\log_{10}$ or $\log_e$, respectively. The latter can also be designated ln.

Logarithm

Since the base for computing the logarithm may typically be either 10 or $e = 2.71828$, it is preferable to indicate common logarithm or natural logarithm, respectively. Alternatively the symbols $\log_{10}$ or $\log_e$ may be used.

Precision

Accuracy and precision are not the same uncertainty measures if there is a *bias* consideration in addition to random effects. When there also can be bias relative to a true value obtained by another means, then an all-inclusive accuracy term should be used rather than precision.

Quality control

Activities of quality control are a subset of those in a broad *quality assurance* program.

Quality assurance

This program to assure a quality product has many features, one of which is *quality control*.

Short axis

This description of an *image* display here is a curtailment of the more rigorous phrase, short axis view.

Standardized uptake ratio

See the commonly preferred synonym, *standardized uptake value*.

Standardized uptake value

Historically, the terms *differential absorption ratio*, *distribution activity ratio*, *differential uptake ratio*, and *standardized uptake ratio*, and their acronyms, have been used instead of the now preferable and synonymous standardized uptake value.

Some detail in how the *region of interest* is geometrically defined should accompany use of the term. Additionally, any alternative that might be used instead of the subject's weight in its calculation should be stated. A good practice often seen is subscripting *SUV* with a descriptor delineating any special methodology used.

It has become universally accepted to give standardized uptake values as numbers without accompanying units of g/ml or kg/l when body weight or lean body mass rather than some other alternative is used in its calculation.

SUR

See the commonly preferred synonym, *standardized uptake value*.

SUV

See *standardized uptake value*.

SUV_{peak}

Accompanying its use, the method for choosing the few *pixels* (*voxels*) whose *activity concentrations* are averaged should be stated. If the method is to use the maximum *pixel* (*voxel*) the preferred term is SUV_{max}.

Vertical long axis

This description of an *image* display here is a curtailment of the more rigorous phrase, vertical long axis view.

Index